HEALTHCARE HEROES

A COMPREHENSIVE GUIDE FOR FUTURE HEALTH PROFESSIONALS

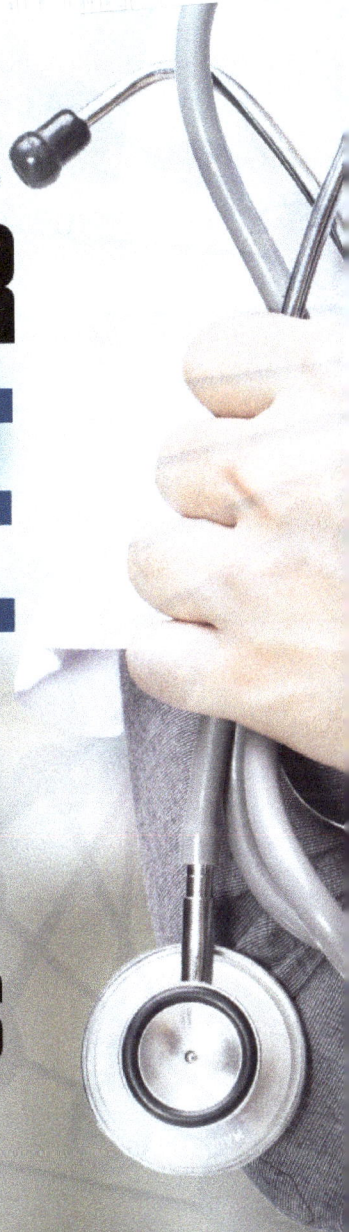

PROF GEORGE ZAFIROPOULOS

Healthcare Heroes:
A Comprehensive Guide for Future
Health Professionals

George Zafiropoulos MSc, MChOrth, DM, MPhil, DiplMEd, FAcadMEd

Consultant Orthopaedic Surgeon, Visiting Professor of University South Wales

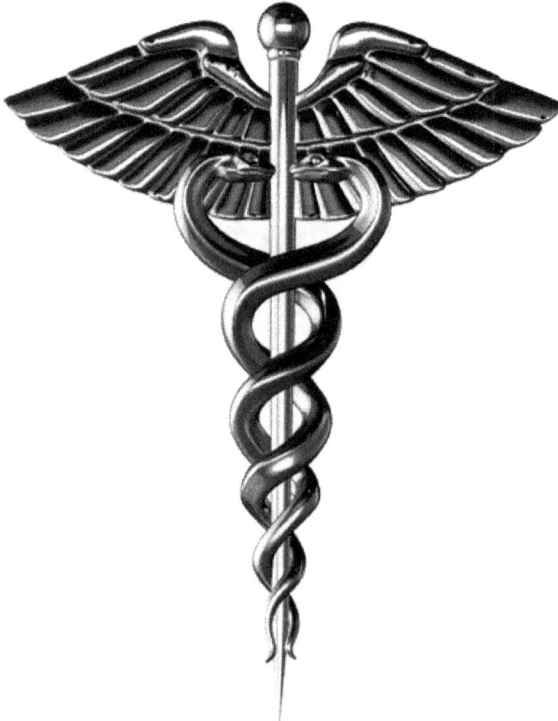

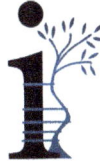

Copyright @George Zafiropoulos

Author: George Zafiropoulos @2024

Title: Healthcare Heroes: A Comprehensive Guide for Future Health Professionals

ISBN: 978-1-0686737-6-4

Category: Health Professionals/ Doctors/ Medical Practitioners

Publisher: Breakfree Forever Publishing

CONTENTS

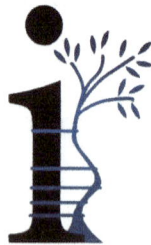

INTRODUCTION

Humans are living in a closed knitted network of contact relationships and supporting each other throughout their existence on this planet. The result of such support is the way they care of each other and their attempt to influence the lives of their close friends as they are trying to make it better.

You may argue that this is not true as wars, crime and a lot of bad is filling human society as these are portrayed in everyday media, but overall the attempt to progress and improvement of life's aspect is the final goal.

Part of this progress is the advancement of natural understanding, science and via this technological improvement. Excluding the "materialistic" way technology can give to humans, the advancement of human thinking, the need of close contact, the understanding of relationships, the attempt to analyse human behaviour were and still are the subject of many studies scholars try to shed light upon.

Part of this constant attempt to understand the surrounding world, as well as themselves, humans observed their environment and the causes life may be cut short. They noted what makes them ill and tried throughout their existence to avoid or change all causes that may lead them to an early loss of their lives.

This is how Medicine was born. It is based on observation and willingness to live.

Becoming a health professional is a very fulfilling profession. You are able to serve people, assist them to become and stay healthy and create the opportunities for them to become positive, productive members of the society. This is an altruistic behaviour health professionals have and they are feeling very proud of the results when they are successful.

Altruism is a natural quality young people have and this is the reason a great number of students are willing to follow the steps and paths of a Health worker.

The following work has been carried out to provide aid to students, their parents and young professionals who wish to follow Medicine or any other Healthcare Studies profession in understanding and explore the qualities a Health Professional has and preparing them for interviews in their field as well as offer guidance in their development so that they are in the best position to present themselves. For the simplicity of the matter, this entire text concentrates on Medicine as a whole, so please feel free to interchange the word "doctor" with any other healthcare profession you may desire. The discussions contained within this work, examples given and opinions expressed are only for guidance, and must therefore be adapted according to individual needs.

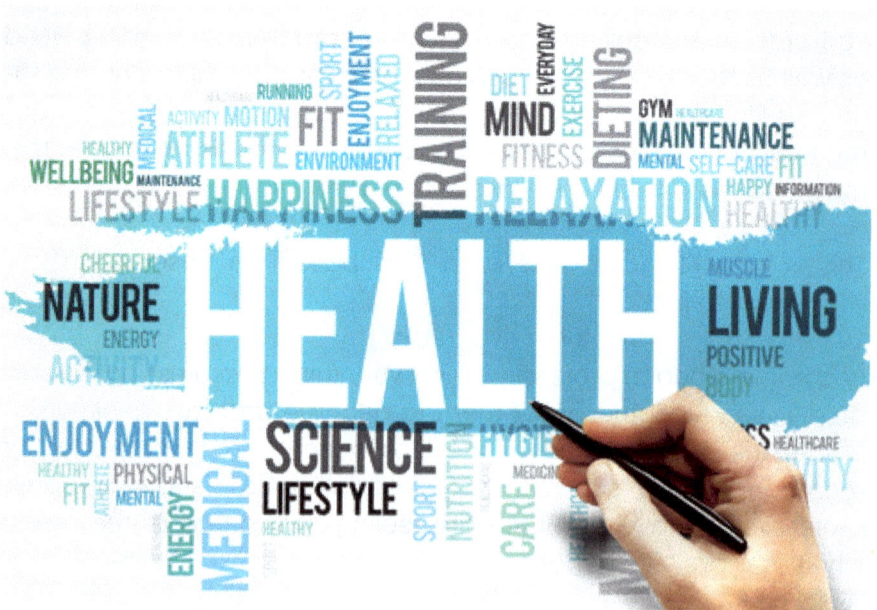

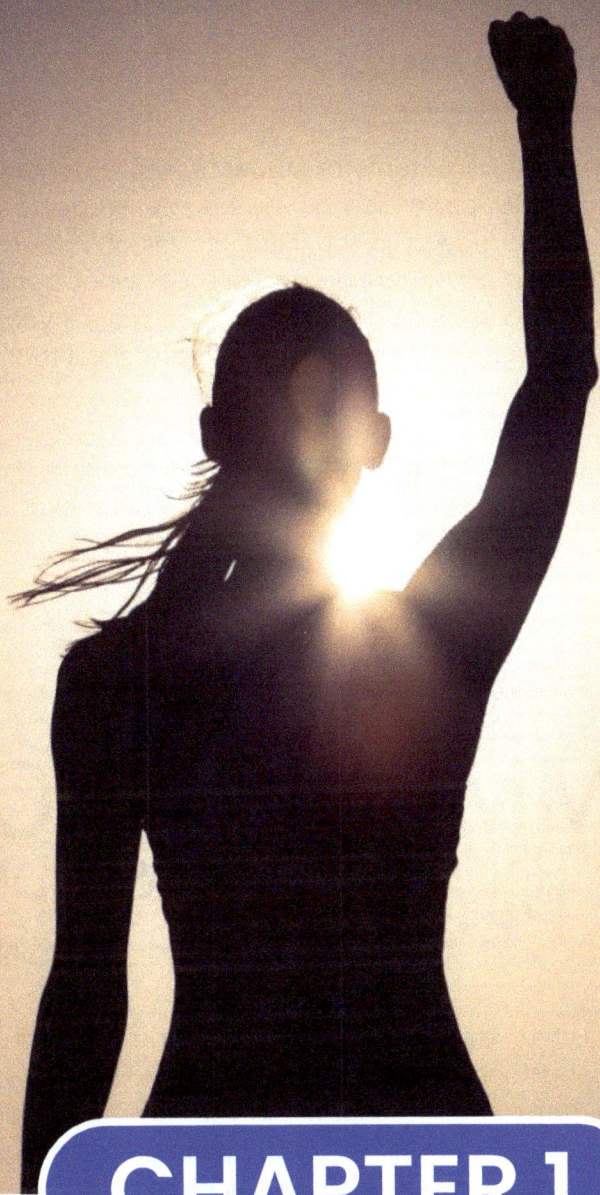

CHAPTER 1

UNDERSTAND YOURSELF

1.1 Knowledge is Power

This is the time you as parents of students who are interested to see them in a health profession or you hopeful students who are either before the College or in the initial stages of your careers in Health care need to pay attention and find out what qualities you have to acquire and what abilities you need to have if you want to be successful within these heart-warming professions that you are dreaming to follow.

You will explore your own abilities, learn how to present yourself to others and find your strengths. These are different for everybody, so be ready to discover yourself.

But first, there is the need to understand the meaning of the words: "information" and "communication". Information is what you give to the people. This is the material which you have, you collect and also pass to others. However, information without communication is not helpful at all. So, what is communication? It is the way you get through to others. It is the way through which you pass on your information. Without communication you do not have any rapport with your "audience". If you are preparing yourself for your life's career, then during an interview or presentation your audience (panel of interviewers) needs to be engaged with you to believe in you and support your position, which will grant you acceptance in their professional family. You may be the best in your field but if you cannot pass this message across to their brains you will fail, as they cannot follow you. This career that you want to follow is your dream, because of this you applied. If you fail you will not able to fulfil this dream.

So, what do you need to do? First of all, prepare yourself for this "battle". Anybody who goes to a "confrontation" needs all the possible weapons as well as defences, to be on their side. Hence, prepare. I know that confrontation is a very strong word, but allow me to use this metaphor to make you understand your position and severity of the entire situation which could lead you to success.

So, what do you need to do? First of all, prepare yourself for this "battle". Anybody who goes to a "confrontation" needs all the possible weapons as well as defences, to be on their side. Hence, prepare. I know that confrontation is a very strong word, but allow me to use this metaphor to make you understand your position and severity of the entire situation which could lead you to success.

- You need to know how to listen, as by listening you will discover your weaknesses and therefore realise what you need to correct. You need to listen to everyone in your environment. This is what some people refer to as a 360 degrees feedback. If you learn how to listen, you can analyse the information given to you and change your behaviour accordingly, as you will now understand what others want from you. You will begin to have a better feel of what the "core" of a question is once presented. Despite this thought you need to be yourself. I know that I said to listen and change, but you must not change your principles, your qualities, your inner world of yours. You are who you are, but you need to focus on your goals and act accordingly. The best term probably is not change but adapt your behaviour, but please do not adapt in a hypocritical way. Do not pretend you are someone else only because you need to reach your goal. Be honest and own the "change" or "adaptation" and make it part of yourself.

- Organise yourself, as this can help you clarify ideas about the subject which you may be negotiating. Organisation also helps in better selection of information. So, what do you need to know first? You are applying to study Medicine. You want to become a doctor. But what do you know about it? How does it feel to be a doctor? You need to know the values of the work, the achievements and goals that you will have in the future, but you also need to find your interests and the skills which you have. Learn as much as you can about Medicine, link with groups of Health workers, listen to their stories, their experiences and the description of their feelings. Allow yourselves to link with the local Hospitals, Health Centres or Surgeries. Visit these places. Spend time within this environment as you will need to know if this is suitable for you. Reflect at the end of every day, on every single information you get and find out if you are fit for this.

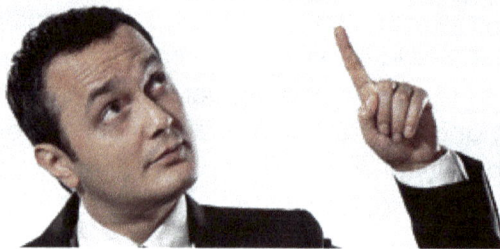

- There are many anxieties in your mind as parent or in your own young mind dear students who wish to follow this line of professions and you are preparing for Medicine. Before we discuss the ways and techniques that you need and must use in an interview for a medical career, you may want to ask yourself if a career in Medicine is the right choice for you in the first place. The following questions are the basic examples to what you should be asking yourself:

Why do I want to become a doctor?

Do I have the qualities of a doctor?

Can I keep dealing, supporting and looking after ill people on a daily basis?

Am I ethical enough to keep practising in medicine, so I can keep secrets?

Can I sustain constant pressure and lifelong training?

Can I sacrifice my personal life with the view of servicing the needs of other human beings while simultaneously fighting for success?

Action

Please try to answer honestly these questions in the best of your knowledge

I will leave you ponder on those before we continue.

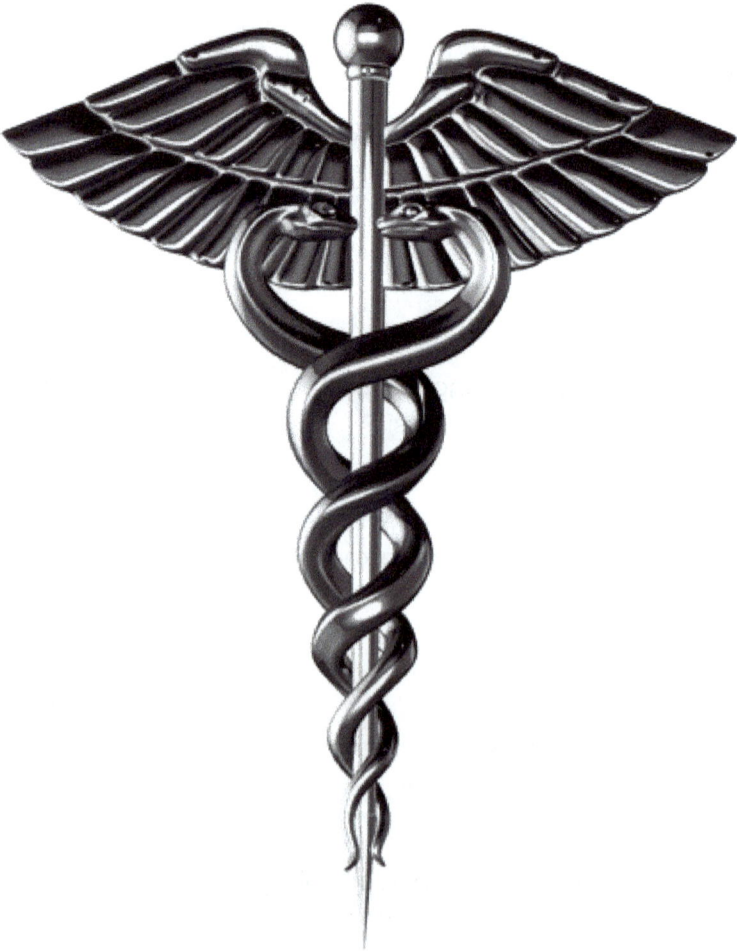

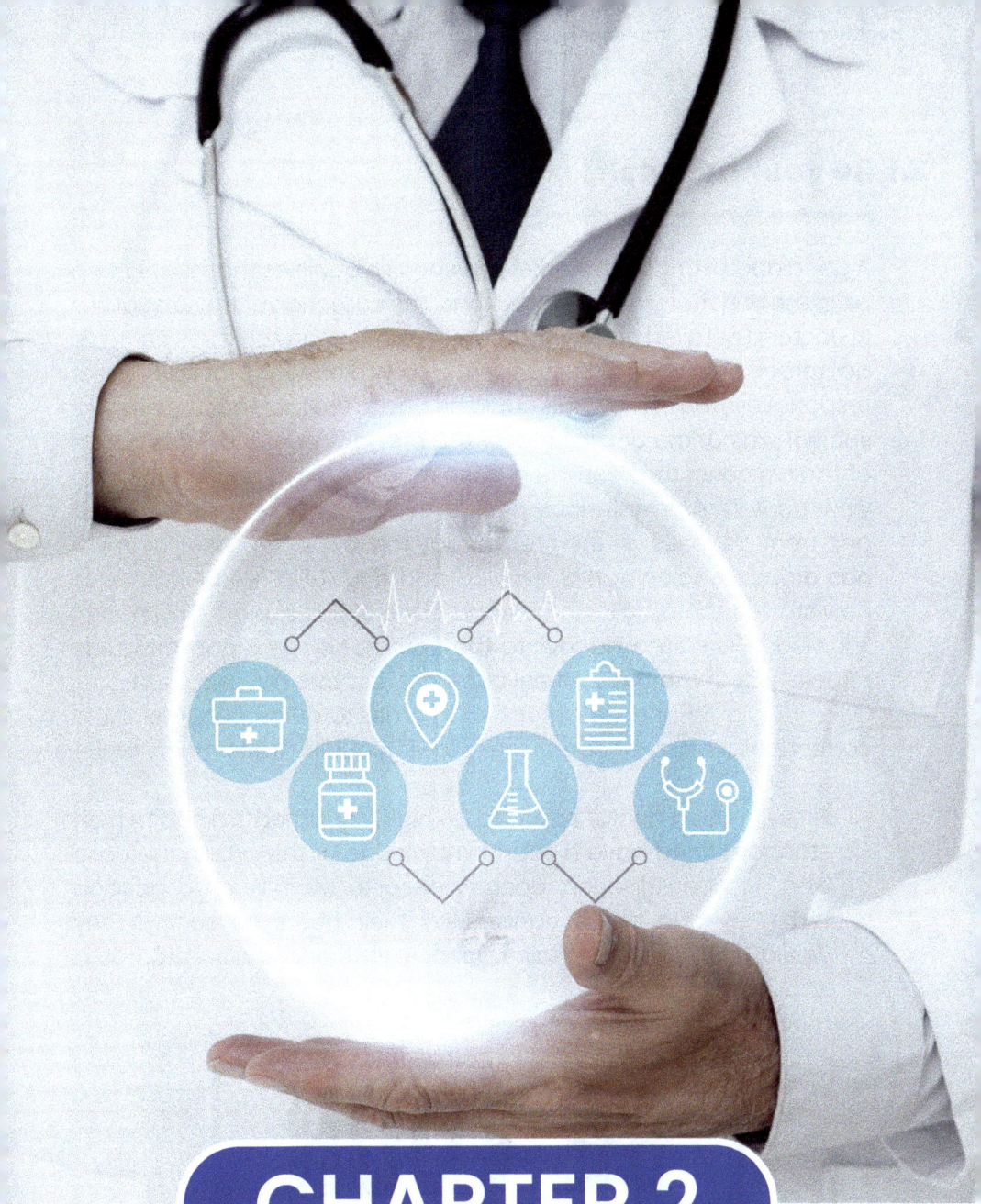

CHAPTER 2

QUALITIES

2.1 Be your best self

A good doctor or health worker has specific qualities that should also be present in many other professions. The collection of these qualities in doctors (detailed below) is necessary since many cultures perceive doctors as being one of the fundamental professions that carry great responsibility. In my view, this could be due to the fact that the healer's subject was of the unknown over the previous centuries. This notion of the unknown that common people had formed caused them to view doctors as mysterious people that were able to understand and treat diseases. In the present day this is not the case, the myth has dropped, science has evolved and a lot of other people have now started to partially understand parts of this subject. This partial knowledge is also a danger to the community as it can misguide people. Within the modern environment, doctors have to be strong, well-articulated and well informed in order to guide patients to the correct path. A doctor needs the following quality traits:

- Firstly, a good doctor needs to be highly qualified, trained to high standards and have a sound knowledge of the art. In the case of a subspecialisation, doctors need to be in such a position that they can be recognised by their peers as such. They would need to be so well trained, that they are accepted as a

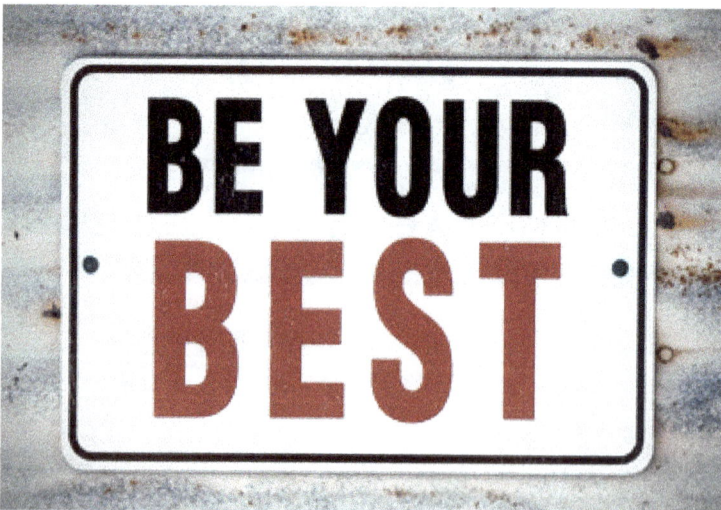

member of their scientific community without any doubt. This ensures the protection of patients from any mistakes and miss-happenings, but must still be able to understand one's own limits. Self-improvement via re-education or continued education is a necessity for one's self and the patients benefit.

- One has to have ownership of their actions and feel pride for the accomplishments made. Dedication to excellence is a requirement in order to achieve self-improvement, with constant work for the betterment of skills and knowledge. By reflecting back, somebody can even learn from unhappy situations such as the loss of a human being, and in this way try to find answers so that this painful experience will not be reiterated.

- A doctor needs to be strong, able to confront difficulties that may scar one's self or others for life and be able to solve problems; to climb and leap over all obstacles, driving patients to the cure and also be able to support patients and their relatives in difficult situations. This inner strength is sometimes not enough and the weight makes doctors, as they are humans themselves, to buckle; but they have to find it back and follow their path if they want to continue practicing.

-

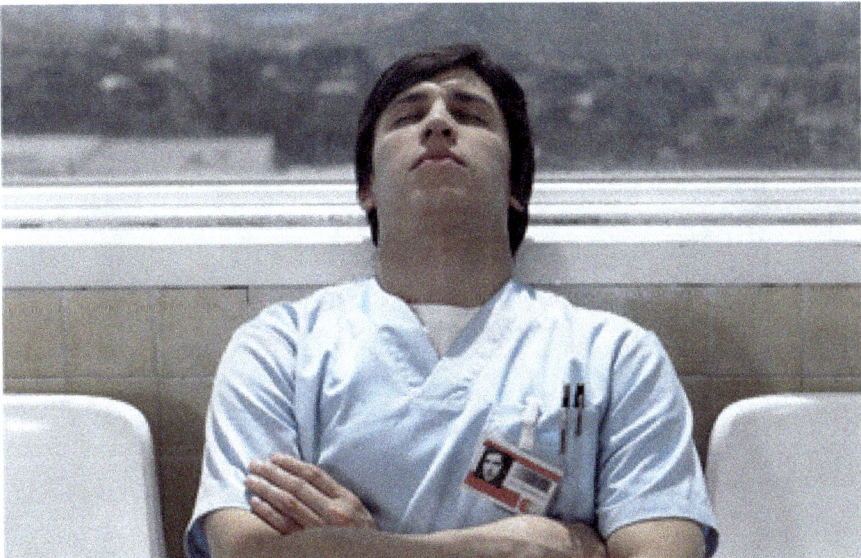

- One needs to be a good communicator, have the ability to simply explain all the complex details of a difficult situation to the patient or family, but has to do this with humble kindness and empathy. Needs to respect the people and be open. This will help not only communication and approachability but also the ability to learn. Doctors can be good communicators by interacting with fellow humans under any circumstances as they need to learn about their patients but it is necessary that doctors have to know about themselves as well as the science which they serve. So, a good doctor has to be able to combine all this for only one benefit; the patient's wellbeing. Having good presence, shows self-respect, this in turn indicates that you also respect other people. So, self-respect is a must if you wish to positively impact people while communicating.

- A good doctor needs to be emotionally stable. During the career, a doctor will confront many cases that are extreme and painful, so it will be necessary to be composed if they wish to be able to resolve these situations. It is not possible for a doctor to run and leave somebody helpless because of an inability to solve the problem within one's own mind. Demonstration of the willingness to help is a necessity. It is not possible to abandon a fellow person in need. It is fare to say that a doctor may need to ask for help from another fellow health professional if they are not expert on the fled, but never leave the patient alone.

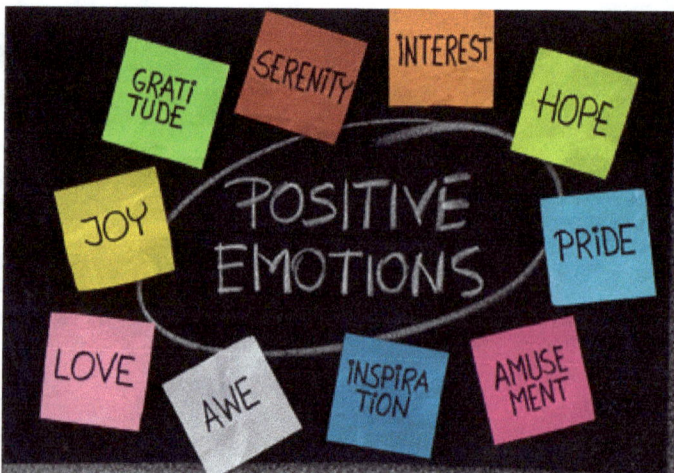

- Compassion, the love to help humanity, a passion and drive for life are all requirements. Needs to have passion for science, for the job, for medicine itself. Needs to be "in love" with Medicine, this is all that he/she has; Medicine. Candidates must be committed to science, to patients and to fellow health professionals; feel responsible for them and their actions, mainly if they are acting under his/her supervision or guidance.

- Patience and the ability to calm patients are key. Patience for the patients who are unable to express themselves, patience for the relatives who are anxious to learn about their loved one's condition, patience for the results of the treatment that are not coming quick enough.

- Doctors have to be able to forgive. Forgiveness for their patient, who is not happy with the outcome of the treatment. Forgiveness for the angry relatives, who have failed to understand the sleepless nights the doctor has spent next to their loved one. Forgiveness about the behaviour of their colleagues, who under stress said inappropriate things, and even forgiveness for themselves, for the time when despite your great efforts, another action may have proven more positive.

- Doctors must be flexible because only this way may they overcome obstacles.

-

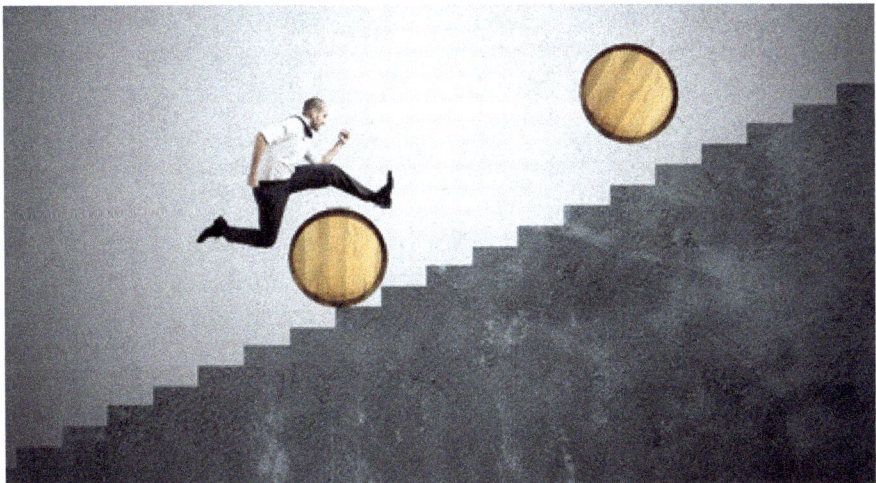

- Doctors need to have endurance. Endurance to leap over the unexpected "fences" and carry on until the next one and the next one and so on. Medicine is sometimes a very sad and lonely job and one needs to acknowledge this. He/she must be like an athlete who runs marathons and despite of the pain, continues; knowing that at the end of the line there is happiness and relief.

- They have to be tolerant; tolerant to everyone who has problems and all who are running towards you, seeking help. Common sense must be applied as this will simplify actions, possibly resulting in better outcomes since everyone will clearly see the situation with great clarity, hence people will not struggle to understand the issues.

- The doctor must be active all the time. Active for the patients, active for the colleagues, active for learning, active for teaching and guiding others. Support must always be provided. Support to patients and their relatives but also to other healthcare workers who are in need of help because they too are in difficulty.

- Confidence is required to take actions but to also remain confident in the made decisions. This enables the patients to gain trust in order to express their condition. Confidence is a double meaning for a doctor and it is necessary to have it. The condition in which the doctors find themselves must be well understood and acted upon accordingly, in a safe way staying committed to the role. In addition, it must not be forgotten that apart from a healer, a doctor is also a teacher, and has to have patience, understanding, commitment, kindness, confidence etc. just as a teacher must. Can it be seen that these teacher qualities are already similar to those of a doctor? Yes, it is clearly evident.

- Observation is a fundamental quality, something doctors had since the beginning of their profession's foundations. Observation of signs and ability to interpret and explain them in a logical fashion, leading to a diagnosis.

- Finally, it is important to have humour. Life is so difficult and the only way to go through it is to have humour. This quality will also be the one that will help everybody; patients, students, colleagues and also doctors themselves to be relaxed. If somebody is relaxed then their performance will be better and safer not only for them but for others too since positivity can be contagious.

So, education, communication, kindness, safety and humour are some of the strongest and most essential qualities without minimising the meaning of all the others. The questions which now have to be answered before the interview techniques for medicine are explored, are:

Can I become a doctor?

Is Medicine for me?

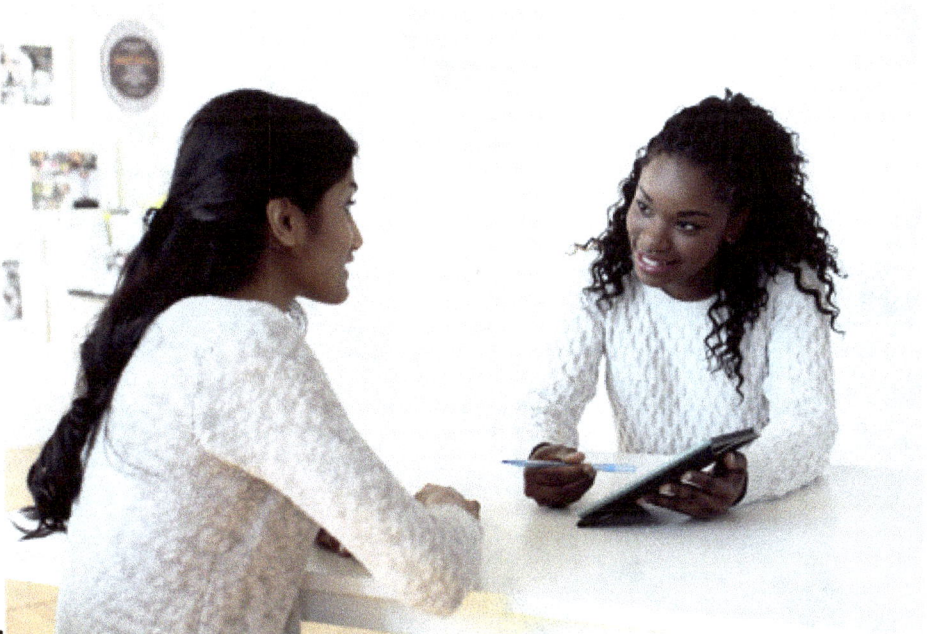

Only after these simple questions are answered truthfully and successfully and the candidate has sought career advice thus understanding the potential limitations, will the candidate be in a position of consent to the Medical Profession.

Action

List how many of these qualities your child, if you are a parent, or yourself have or if you think that you can develop them.

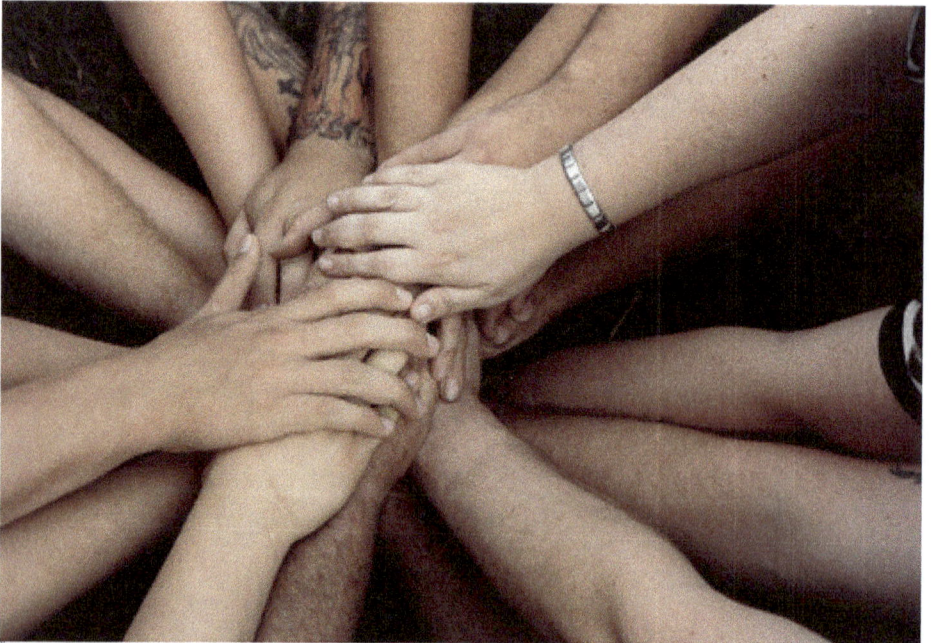

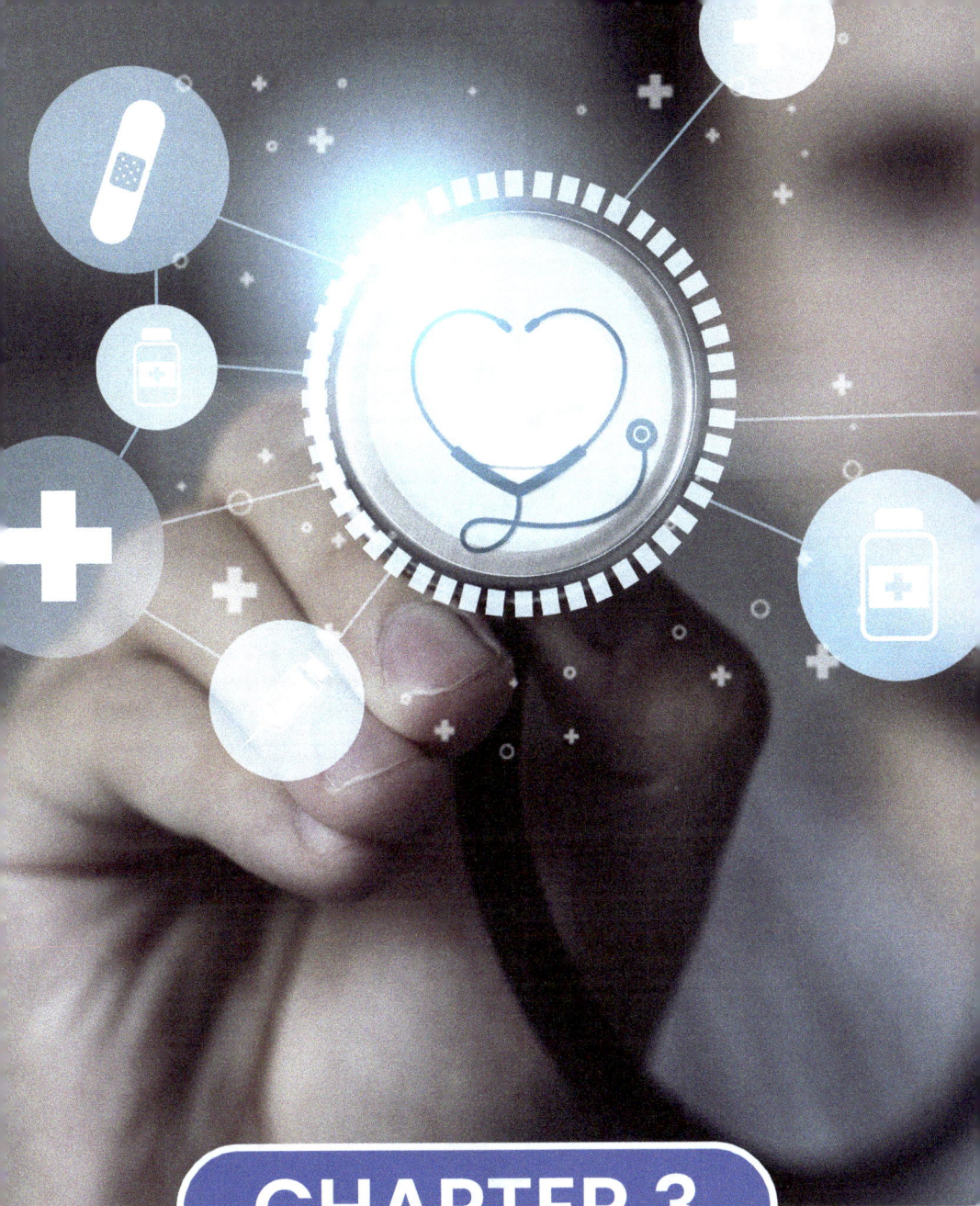

CHAPTER 3
PREPARE YOURSELF

3.1 Ready, Steady, Go

Following this "brainstorm" and the questions associated with this, you need answers to satisfy the questions that are now flooding your mind. You need to analyse them and prepare further. You should research about the course, organisation or job/position that you applied for, the University/Institution and the reasons that drove you to select all these. You also need to write about yourself in relation to Medicine and the University. This is your first communication step with others. You need to be selected out of hundreds of applicants who applied for the same position and you have to stand out in front of all the others. As you already know, people constantly move. They are part of the universal traffic that takes them from one part of their lives to another. But just as on motorways, cars move in different lanes, the same happens with people. You must be prepared to travel in the fast lane, as this way you will overtake all the others and become more successful. There is this statistical analysis based on Pareto 20:80 ration indicating that only 20% of the applicants will go through. Become one of them.

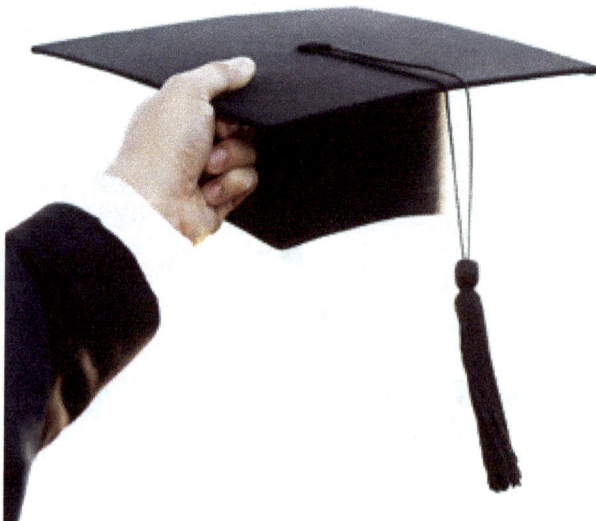

The fuel you have is the preparation and knowledge which you accumulate and this is going to push you forwards. GO FOR IT!!!! This translates to you now having to write your Curriculum Vitae (CV), Resume and/or Personal Statement. You can give any name you want to it but it is the same overall philosophy, sell yourself and stand out. But how can you write an interesting summary of yourself? The majority of the people are very "confused" when it comes to writing about themselves. We are educated in such a way that we must avoid promoting ourselves. It is taken as "selfish", "egotistical", "arrogant" and "impolite". Someone who "blows their own trumpet" is considered to be pompous and rude. This is the difficulty that all have when the time comes to write a CV. The attempt is to learn how to write one, and my first piece of advice is to be honest. The panel will ask personal questions, so if you are not honest, they will find out, and believe me they can. The first tip for your Interview Technique for Medicine is HONESTY.

3.2 Curriculum Vitae

To get a feel of how to part-write your CV, you can see some made up examples in the appendix, but please do not copy them, as these are not going to help you, because these are not YOU. You have to write about yourself, do not forget it. The examples are only giving you some stimulus to surface some of your deep existing experiences which you forgot about. Please take them as stimuli, not as copies that can drive you to success. If the CV is not based on you, you will fail. As already mentioned, be HONEST. Despite the fact that you initiated the making of your CV, do not forget that the first ever communication to the others is through your application. You have to be clear, concise and the presentation must be immaculate. The writing needs to be simple and has to make sense. The CV will then follow whereby the same process has to be carried out. In addition to honesty, you need to be able to write clear, sensible statements that are to the point. The best application can only be achieved through concentration therefore think positive. Be serious about your application. Keep your writing and layout tidy, clear and easy to understand. Take your time for preparation, but please do not submit it late. The application has to be submitted on time as every institution, organisation and University requests. Make sure that all the information you include is real, true and up to date. Show your motivation and pay attention to the detail and quality of information which you give out. If you have done any apprenticeships in connection to Medicine, write about them. This application IS ABOUT YOU. Do not forget this. Be clear. Be serious. Be honest. Be presentable. Be motivated. Be positive.

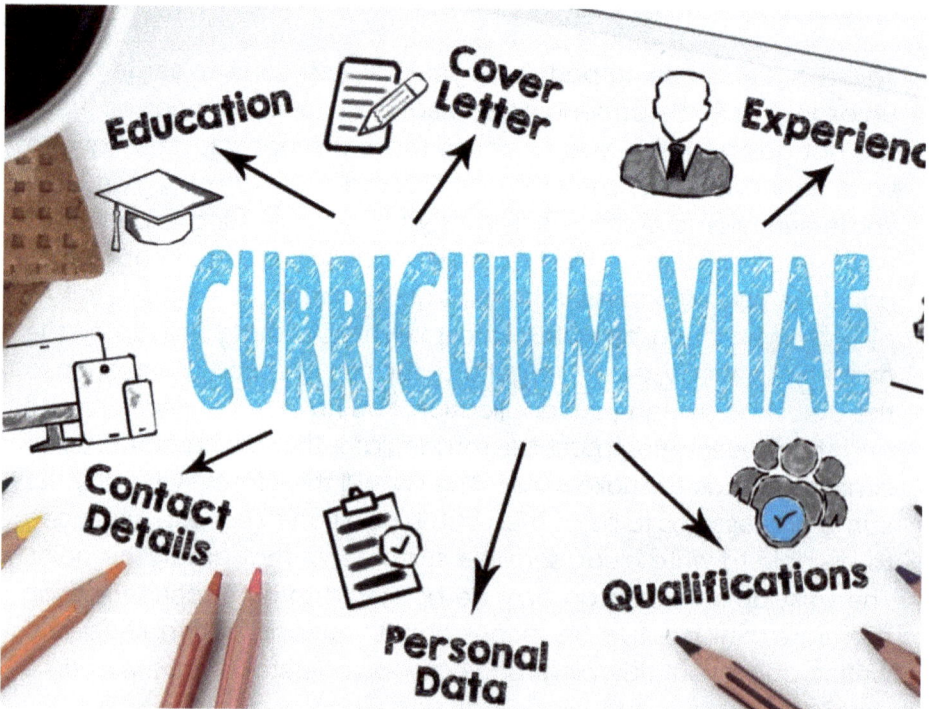

3.3 Presentation

The interview is all about how you present yourself, this time it is not about you, but how the others will perceive you and receive your presentation. This is about them and how they will understand you. Imagine yourself in the interview room. You never thought about it but now your anxiety is sky high. Remain calm and control yourself. Before you do anything, control your emotions. Analyse the time of the day. If for example, it is nearly noon you have to adjust yourself to it. Are you the first or the last candidate? How many times has the panel heard the same stories? Are they hungry? You must take all this into consideration so this way you can control yourself, your timing, your style and you can show to them that you respect them. A small quiet initial statement such as "I will not keep you long; I am mindful that lunchtime is fast approaching…" may be to your favour. Do not overdo it though, as they may think that you are in a hurry. If you can, try to find out who will be present in the panel. This way you may prepare yourself better, knowing the potential likes and dislikes of the people who will be in front of you, assessing your personality, character, knowledge and experience. You should not start talking before you are in control of your emotions and also understand their emotional status. All this analysis has to take seconds, not hours. Do not forget that if they are tired, they may be distracted so may not listen to you, therefore keep answers simple. Some call this "framing of your statement". What is the meaning of it? Let's say that you are in a gallery. If you observe, the different pictures/paintings have different frames and the two parts (picture and frame) will react with each other emphasizing the area of the picture or some colours of it in the way that the artist or the art gallery owner wants you to see. The same technique should be used during the interview. There is the possibility that one question, despite that you felt you answered correctly, lost its track. Reframe it. Explain the same thing in a different manner so this way you clarify the subject and you pass the message through. Do not forget that the main goal here is for you to successfully go through to the Medical School or get that job. This is the picture, the goal and you have to frame it in the best frame you have, even if you have to change a dozen of different ones around. You follow the goal and manipulate everything in such a way that you use the best tools and the best products for the construction of your frame. This picture has to be desirable, sought after and easily sellable. Even in the rare possibility that one of the interviewers is confrontational with you, you follow the same technique. Keep calm, listen, and do not react with emotions, instead reframe and sell. This is the way to success.

For a successful interview you have to be prepared, do your groundwork. Find out all that you can about your course, University or organisation. I advise you to go to open days before the interview. This knowledge will control your emotions, your anxiety and will open yourself to the audience. You must remember that openness leads to relaxation and relaxation to better results, as all this reflects onto your panel. Remember something that has been previously mentioned. The whole point of your presentation is not about you, but about the picture that the others will create about you when they see and understand you. It is known that approximately 70% of the interview is won or lost as soon as you have entered the room. They can make up their mind in the first 30 seconds if you are somebody who is suitable for them or not. This is in relation to the way that you present yourself. Make yourself look professional. If you pass this step, this is the time that the panel will now listen to you. Do not damage this initial appearance of yourself; try to pass this test. Do not underestimate the panel's intelligence, so you must not lie, trick them, or any sort of playing around, as they will "punish" you and move your dream that little bit further away. Try to reflect and evaluate your position at all times. Be alert, yet pleasant. When you present yourself, you have to be a clear picture of yourself, acceptable to enter the organisation or institution which you are planning to go to. This institution is the Medical School and the organisation is the professional body and family of the doctors. You must be well dressed and presentable with suitable attire. There is a dress code and you must adhere to it. Many interviewers choose and decide upon first impressions, so dress accordingly. You must dress smart and clean. The Medical School will not accept anyone who is dressed inappropriately, with unhealthy body odour, or alternatively somebody who is dressed too "loud".

3.4 Appearance

Hair should be well combed or casually styled as opposed to inappropriately styled. Your presentation is the most important thing as this is your first impression to the panel and it defines you. You have to have clean clothes in addition to your clean, polished shoes. Please do not present yourselves wearing trainers. Avoid trainers, even if you feel comfortable in them. Clothes have to be classic and preferably dark in colour, mainly if you apply to old traditional institutions.

For the ladies the dress code is; no short skirt or short dress; conservative outfit. Avoid low cut tops, short dresses with the whole back exposed and red or lilac shoes. Women should be well presented, with well attended nail polish, if this is necessary or appropriate. Remember your hair must be well combed. Inappropriate hair styles are certainly not popular in front of an interview panel, particularly ladies wearing excessive hair accessories.

For the gentlemen, white or light-coloured shirts with a classic, darker low motif tie (either mono-coloured or with light minimal stripes) that matches the colour of the suit. The preferred colours are blue, brown or beige. The clothes need to be conservative but comfortable. Avoid wearing large collared, colourful patterned and un-tucked shirts. Avoid ties with printed characters on them or wearing weighted jewellery. You are not in a party but in an interview. All this is unacceptable. Men should be well groomed.

At the pictures above you can see appearances you must avoid

If you carry papers with you, they should preferably be contained in a dark organised folder that is labelled so that they are easily accessible if proven to be necessary. A last-minute search followed by the comments "I don't believe it, I am sure I had placed it here..." is not acceptable. Some of the interviewers do not wish to see any documentation as all the information has already been represented in your CV, but what if they would like to see any official documents

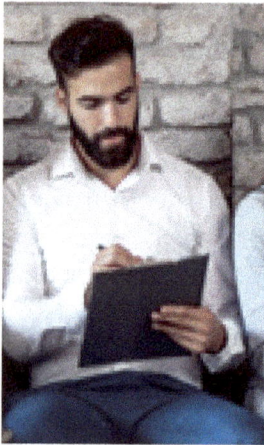

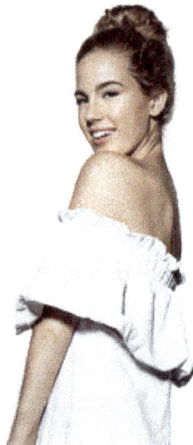

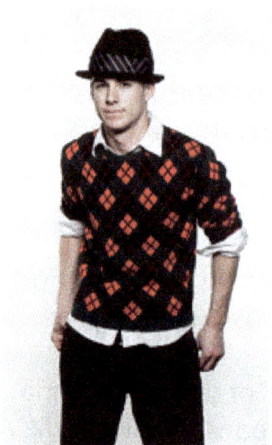

or certifications? Do not rely on the "they will not ask" option. Be prepared and show them how well organised you are. This is a bonus point.

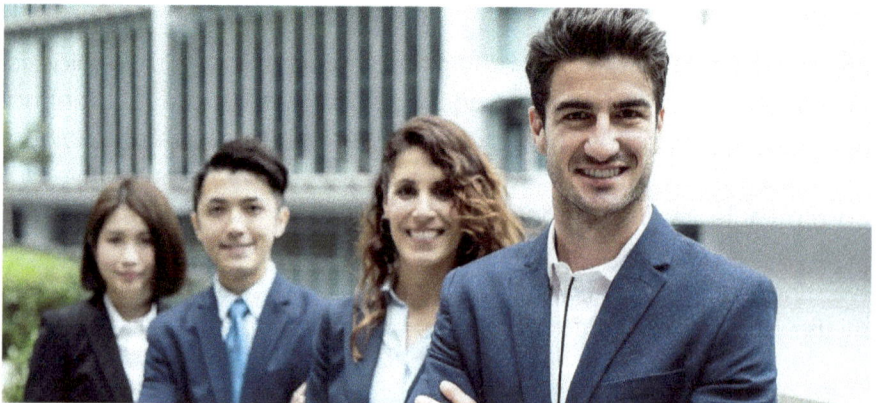

3.4.1 Hygiene & Foundation

You have to be clean, so a shower or bath prior to the interview is essential. A very important point; body odour, due to the food you may have consumed the previous day. For example, you may need to go for an interview to another city which will be held early in the morning. For this reason you may decide to travel and arrive at the destination the previous day to stay at a local hotel. At dinner time you may want to go to a restaurant that is usually recommended by the hotel's receptionist. You should avoid consuming any food that could possibly produce any unpleasant body odour the following morning, which will come out with your body perspiration. Do not forget that you will be anxious and anxiety creates this perspiration effect on our bodies. Please avoid these foods and try to eat something neutral, but please eat. If you starve yourself, it could be a disaster. You need glucose to function and if the glucose levels are low, you will be hungry as well as irritated. So, eat but eat neutral. I would also recommend eating your morning breakfast. By holding your glucose levels correctly, you will be alert, happy, relaxed and you will have better chances for success. The perfume you may wear needs to be light and neutral. Remember you are going to an interview not a date. You have to smell clean and fresh. Do not force the panel to open the windows. Heavy perfume and perspiration are a very bad combination. Do not underestimate perspiration, because it will be there. It is a natural process, at least for the initial moments of the interview.

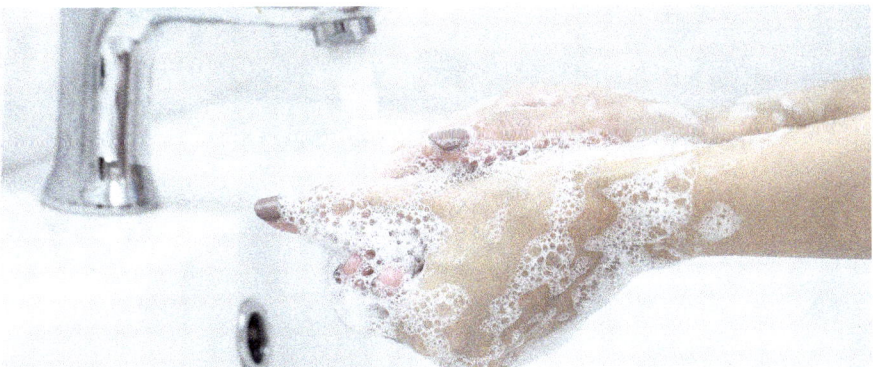

3.5 Keeping Calm

Many people believe that courage and confidence is only accessible or produced through other means and not by themselves, so they consume plenty of alcohol, emptying bottles prior to the interview. This is unacceptable and most unprofessional. Do not consume any alcohol. This has the following bad effects on you. Firstly, smells and think the advice I just gave you about body odours above. Secondly and most importantly, alcohol obscures your mind. In an interview you need to have a clear mind so you can understand the questions fully, articulate the answers and give them to the panel. You need to have the ability to reframe the answer if the vibes of the panel are not the expected ones as mentioned before. How can you do all this complicated mind process if your brain is under the shadow and influence of alcohol? You will not be able to control your mind which will result in you losing your potential position and failing your interview. You would have kicked your dream to the curb. Courage by the use of alcohol is not courage, it is a disaster. True confidence comes from your preparation and your knowledge of the subject. It comes from within yourself and it's the reflection of your confidence which will mask your anxiety, the feeling of intimidation and fear that you have in your mind. The equation is, preparation produces confidence which creates the win over anxiety. The serenity of the mind is an internal control which does not need any help from external sources. Something that helps bring relaxation is a prompt arrival at the institution.

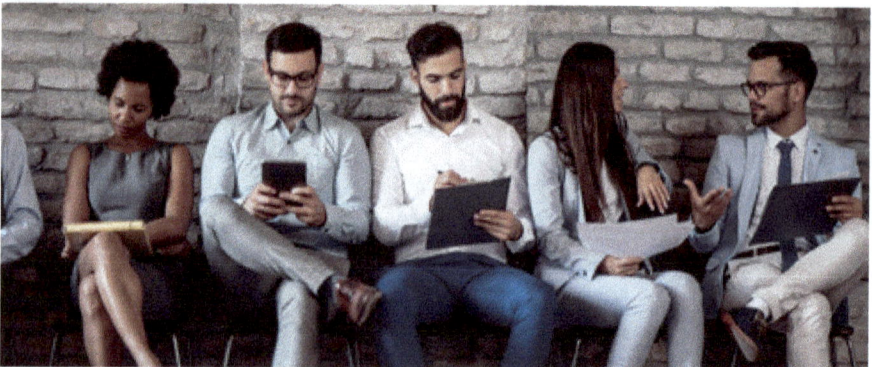

Give at least 30 minutes to yourself to be within close proximity of the interview area. Late public transport, roadworks/diversions and so on are no excuses. There are the following benefits for this action:

Firstly, you accommodate yourself with the surroundings.

You show that you are organised, punctual and professional.

You can once more see the environment which you may have experienced when you visited the place during the University open day or previous meeting/visit. This can bring back memories, discussions of that day or experiences that you had at that time which you may have forgotten.

You may have the opportunity to meet some of the important old/current students or employees already there and ask them important questions which you have just thought of as you consider these people important. Such a discussion may be somewhat therapeutic to your mental status and decrease the levels of anxiety because the other person will give you an "air" of re-assurance.

You may have brief contact with other members of the staff such us secretaries of the institution, who believe me understand the stress you are under. With their soft words and discussions this may help reduce your adrenaline levels.

Some say that as a candidate you should stay standing in the waiting room, because this way you demonstrate that you are energetic and enthusiastic while others say that you should sit down to show you are calm and confident. In my humble opinion please sit down. This way you will stay relaxed and put your thoughts into perspective. Additionally, allow me to use the following metaphor. Visualise the institute as a suit, or a pair of shoes. You have "tried it/them on" during the open day and you liked it/them. But now you have to wear it/them. Any new suit or pair of new shoes gets more comfortable the more times you wear it/them. So, give yourself time and "wear the University". Get into the environment and feel warm and accepted. This will help you relax as you will feel calm. Ultimately, this comfort will then help you reach the next step. The next step is entering the room where the panel awaits; the interview room. If you truly feel comfortable, there is nothing else apart from this one step. These people in there are not spitting fire dragons, they are people like you. They are not the bullies of the next neighbourhood who will not play with you and push you around. They will not eat you alive. The only thing that they want is to select the best for their school, and they think that you could potentially be that person. After all, the reason you are sat in front of them right now is because they are interested in you and liked the initial contact you had with them. They have positive thoughts about you. They want you but you need to prove that their gut feeling was right. When you are relaxed, comfortable and happy, they will get these positive vibes and they will "play with you" in their own field or neighbourhood. They will also listen to you and allow you to present your rules.

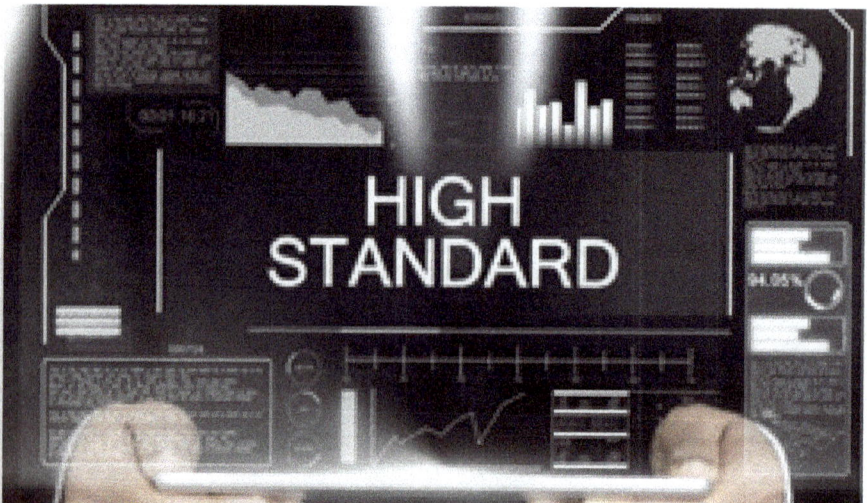

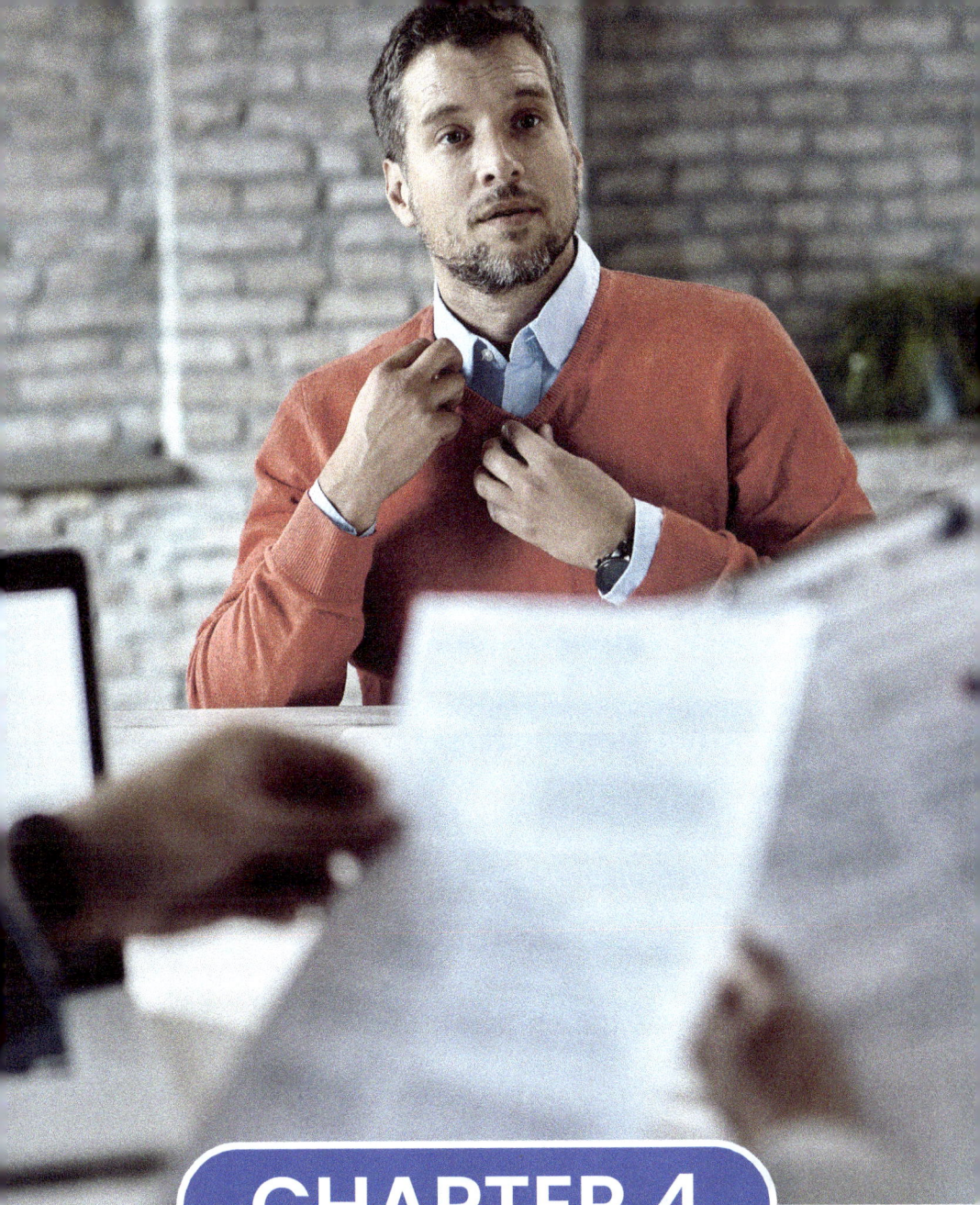

CHAPTER 4

THE INTERVIEW

A typical interview will be structured in the following summarised way:

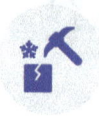

Both yourself and the panel participate in Ice-Breaking & Greeting

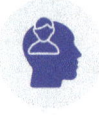

They ask you character & personality-based questions

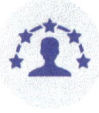

They ask you experience-based questions

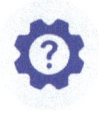

They ask technical-based questions

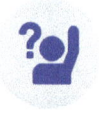

You ask them any questions

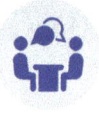

End of interview

Not all interviews are the same however and the order may vary, however the overall structure will always remain. So, let's dive deeper and go through these below.

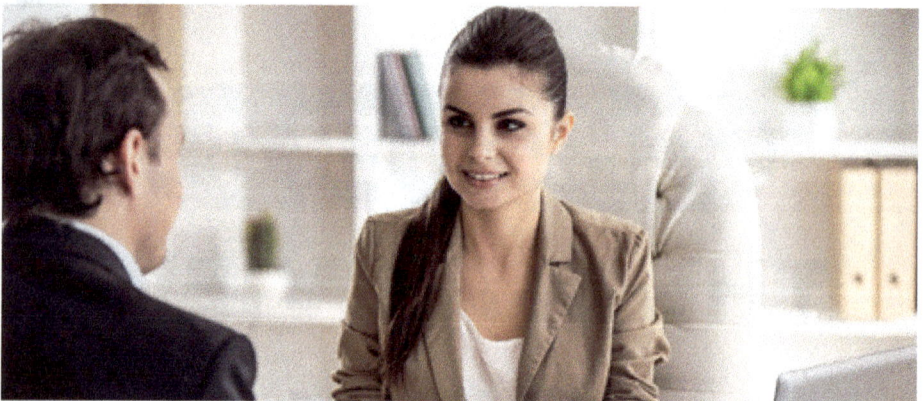

4.1 First Impression

As you enter the interview room, the interviewers/panel will firstly look for your positive presentation, posture and body language. Yes, you are entering in their room, their field, but do not be afraid or intimidated. They will smile at you as they want to make you feel comfortable; but you already know that comfort and confidence comes from within yourself. Now show this with the following:

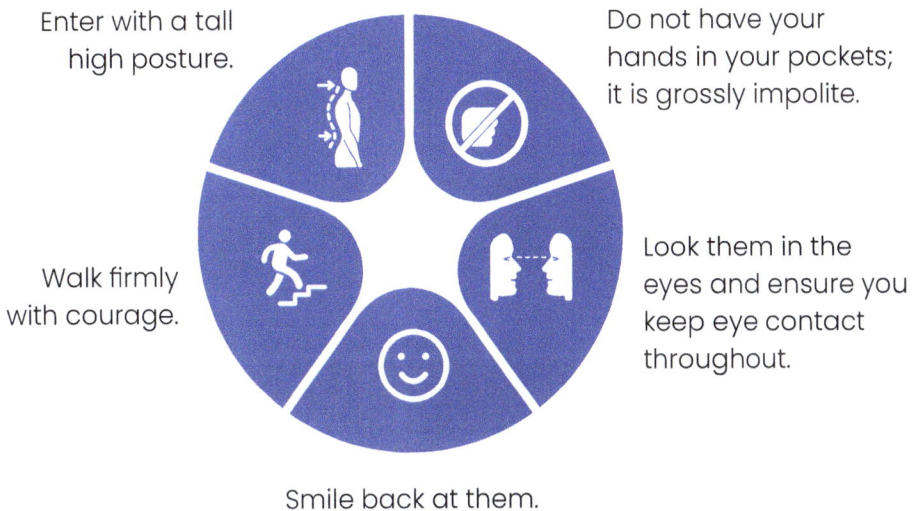

Enter with a tall high posture.

Do not have your hands in your pockets; it is grossly impolite.

Walk firmly with courage.

Look them in the eyes and ensure you keep eye contact throughout.

Smile back at them.

Doing the above has a double effect. The panellists see your smiley face and they see that you are courageous since eye contact is the first part of communication. As they communicate with you, take the opportunity to get know them a little. You may now be wondering how and if this is even possible to be done in these split seconds? The answer is yes, it can be done in split seconds. You will recognise from their eyes who is the possible friendly person or the confrontational person or even the sceptical one about you. This way you can prepare yourself and recognise your opponents. Do not forget, they will try to establish a rapport with you and you should try to do the same. So, let it happen. If it is possible to shake their hands do it. In most instances this happens anyway, but make sure that your hand is not sweating, as this will reveal your anxiety status. The hand shake has to be firm, not soft and weak but not overpowering to the extent that you crush their hands. If you give a weak handshake the panel members may take it as insecurity. On the other hand, if you crush their hands, then it can be taken by some as an intimidating gesture and they may change their approach to you. If the desk is too wide and you cannot reach them for a hand shake, you just make a polite acknowledgement gesture with your head, looking each and every member of the panel straight into their eyes with a smiling face. Remember what I said, a polite gesture using your head. Do not stretch your arm above your head as the next president of a country or salute with a military-like salute, neither uses the words "hi dudes...", even if you saw this at the latest blockbuster film. This is not appropriate at all. If you do so they will look at you as an alien person and they will block their minds for the rest of the interview. They will not listen to anything you say even if you are a genius of the whole universe. Effectively, you would have failed before you began. You would have failed yourself.

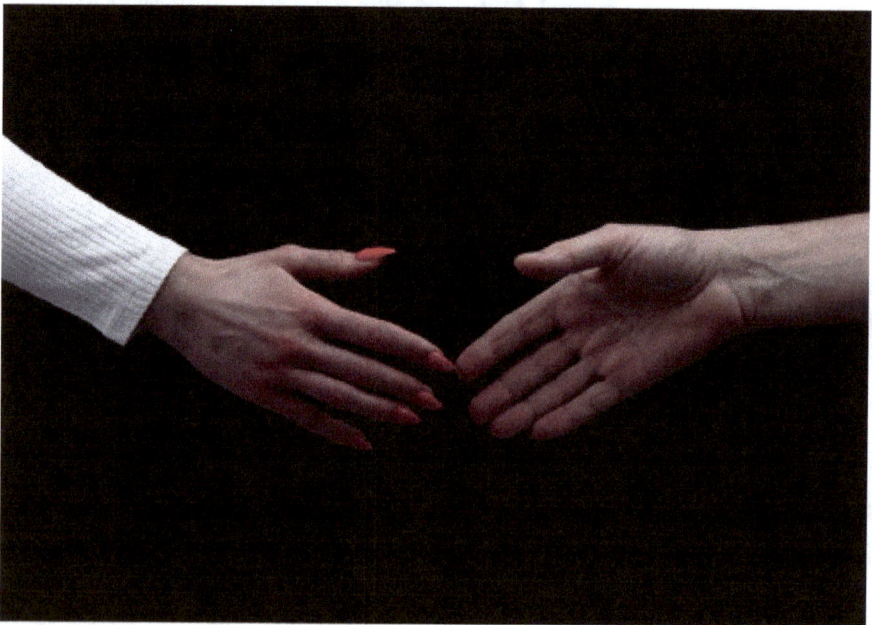

4.2 Control

You will be indicated to take a seat, usually opposite the panel. Do not sit before you are told to do so. In all cases keep the eye contact with the panellists and smile. Do not forget communication commenced upon the entrance to the room.

Place your folder preferably next to your chair if the folder is large or the desk small, otherwise you can place it on the table next to you, however it is best placed next to your chair. The reason is so that you do not distract the panel members with foreign objects, thus giving you their undivided attention. There are further things you also need to consider:

- Do not sit on your hands.

- Do not keep your hands under the table, leaning your body forwards. This may come across as being nervous. Sit proud, upright and calmly with your hands on the table.

- Likewise, do not sit back in an extra-relaxed casual manner. Slouching or resting on the side of the chair may come across as if you do not care.

- Do not fidget with your hands or any other objects. What do I mean by saying this? Do not play with your pen and paper for example. Do not fiddle with your fingers. Keep them together perhaps with your hands touching, but not interlocked fingers or crossed arms. You do not want to come across as someone who thinks is higher than the interviewers.

- Hands can very easily show your feelings and if you are nervous this can become evident. Therefore, control your finger and hand motion as you do not want to show panellists you are nervous.

- When outside or even inside the interview room (this is worse) do not tap on the table to a tune fixed in your mind using your fingers or a pen as if you are trying to meditate and forget your sorrows and stress.

- Try not to bounce or shake your leg under the table.

- Keep calm.

If you have practised pre-interview techniques at home with your friends or relatives then I am sure that you will not be nervous so you shouldn't have anything to worry about. Pass this message to them, "I am not nervous".

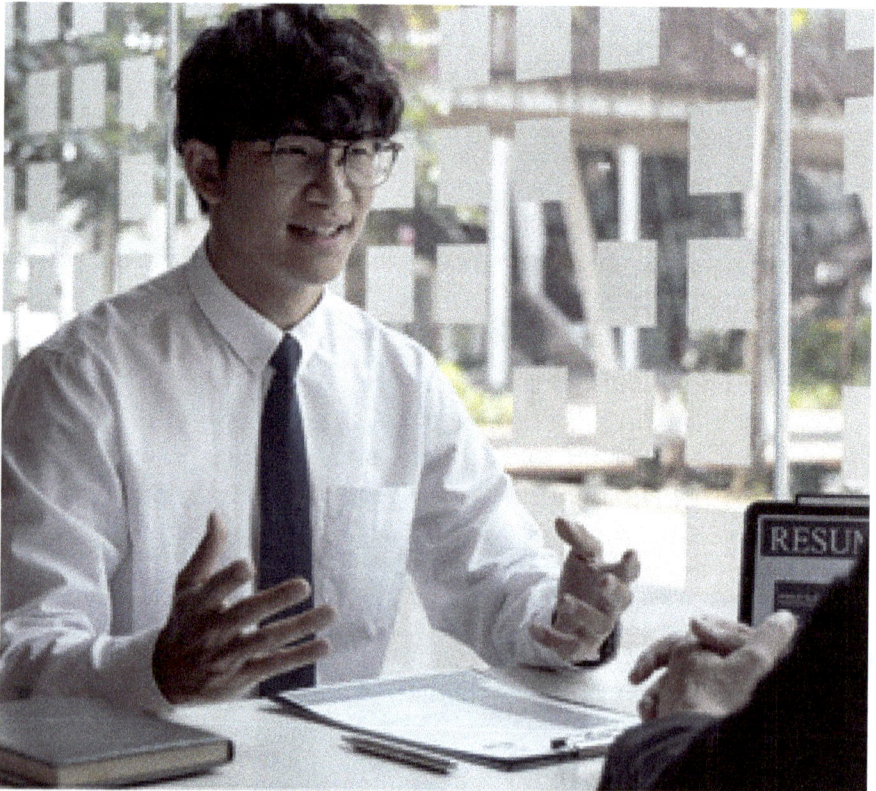

4.3 The Small Talk

To begin with, the panellists usually incorporate an "ice breaking" period or conversation, so they may talk to you about the weather, the experiences that you had in town, if you had trouble finding them, if you are local or not, what is your favourite food or even what the name of your pet is. Use this opportunity to your advantage and show them how friendly, polite and easy to talk to you are, they will like you for it, especially if you can find any common interests. Do not be afraid to ask them questions too, but do not aim to their personal life. They will see you are a proactive and engaging person.

4.4 The Hot-Seat

When they ask you a question, do not rush to answer before the question is finished and has been asked. Keep listening to understand the depth of the question and also what parts can you extract from this to use in your answer. Do not worry too much, the question is not like a mathematical problem whereby all the parameters are given and there is only one clear outcome. In mathematics the outcome is usually one and unique. This is not the case for interviews and will not be what you confront. Usually there is more than one answer therefore the outcome depends on which path you take. This is usually the answer which is more convenient to you. The questions are usually open as the panel wants to help you develop and unfold yourself in front of them, showing them how well you can work with them in the future, showing them your ethics, integrity, etc. But be careful how you perform the unfolding. You must not leave yourself open to any attack. I said unfold, not expose. Always keep answers clear, concise, to the point and relatable to the question. Do not waffle, but do not be vague either. Give them enough to chew on so they can perhaps ask more if they are interested to go deeper.

By the end of the interview you may have to answer specific or technical questions. Even with these questions you can still find a way to answer in a brief manner while still providing them with the answer they are looking for. Difficult? That is why it is important to play a pre-interview game with friends, in order to practise. But be careful to avoid the so called "cultural noise". What is this? It is when you listen to other opinions and thoughts too much before the interview or during your preparation, resulting in answers that to do not represent yourself. These are usually responses you give to try and be socially acceptable and fit in with the crowd. Please try to avoid this as you may end up not answering the question at all. This may be because you do not have an answer. What I mentioned before is to answer the question in a way that will not lead them to hurt you, that is if you believe or are afraid that this can happen. Answer the points of the question. You are not discussing melons when they are asking you about lemons just because both are yellow in colour and share the same letters. If you genuinely do not know the answer, just say so rather than create a story of your own. You will give them the certainty that you are honest and they will appreciate your courage to point out a potential weakness of yours. This will give you time to recuperate and fight for another question. Make sure that the words which you say are clear and well understood. Do not lose yourself in a labyrinth of sentences. Sentences must be short and to the point. As somebody in the past said to me "grab the bull by the horns". This is a clean move to defeat the bull as you are straight to the point. I know that you would have practised some of the questions at home. You can also find some commonly referred questions and answers later on to help and guide you. I stress the word guide. This is because you must not memorise answers as this can come across as robotic. You need to know questions. Every one of you is a separate individual from all the others with different experiences, so you cannot have the same answer to the question. If you try to memorise the answer and you forget a word then this can cause you problems as you may fail to answer the question. You have to be natural. Answers have to be naturally produced. Practise the questions and discuss the answers, but remember this is an interview and not a poem contest in which you have to say the poem word by word. You are not someone else or a parrot. Remember the process of the answer and the facts of the answer must be, I stress again, exclusive to you.

4.5 Charisma- It doesn't end at "First Impressions"

When you are answering the questions keep on smiling and looking at them straight in the eyes. You know, smiling is not a permanent frozen position of your mouth and face, trying to imitate Mona Lisa. Smiling is also a feeling and this can very easily be seen in the eyes, easier than you think. The eyes can smile while the mouth talks. Only after the sentence and talking have finished the smile returns to the mouth. Practise this at home, using all the available people, relatives, neighbours or friends as the members of the panel. With this practise you have the cognition to use the same technique with the interviewers. One common trick is to look yourself in the mirror and practise. This is the "mirroring" technique. Observe all your expressions and correct them. Originally, look at the person who made the question, but when answering keep looking at all of them. Eye contact is key. You need to build a rapport with them. As you can see, no matter how many times this has been stated previously, preparation is paramount and can eliminate your anxiety.

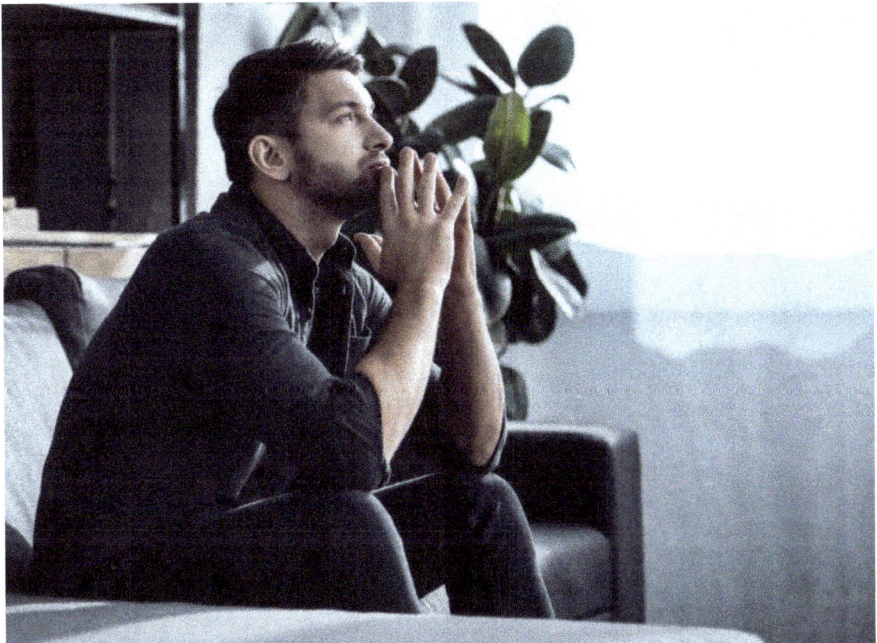

4.6 Body Language- Half way there, don't stop now!

Just because you are likeable, you have come across genuine and a real potential asset to the institution/practice so far, it does not mean you need to relax, become laid back in your approach and forget about everything we have discussed so far just because you think you have this one in the bag already. Do not assume. As you sit there in front of the panel, you can't help but feel stressed at times. This is natural and gets easier with time (and yes you guessed it, preparation/practise, get the picture?). You need to feel comfortable, but please do not slouch, lean back and cross your legs or spread yourself across multiple seats. Yes, you have to be in comfort but really you are also participating in an interview, you are not on holidays sipping a piña colada and neither are you on a cruise laying on a lounger next to the pool enjoying the sun. Comfort means, the relaxation of your mind. The current distressful status you are in at this stage should not be reflected as disrespectful behaviour towards others by the position of your body. Can you see how body language is important and how it can make or break you? When somebody says to you be comfortable it does not mean that you have to be arrogant or aggressive towards them. Be careful as your posture and actions can reveal your feelings and your personality. What is the correlation between postures and state of mind that your body can reveal? Here are some of the most common ones:

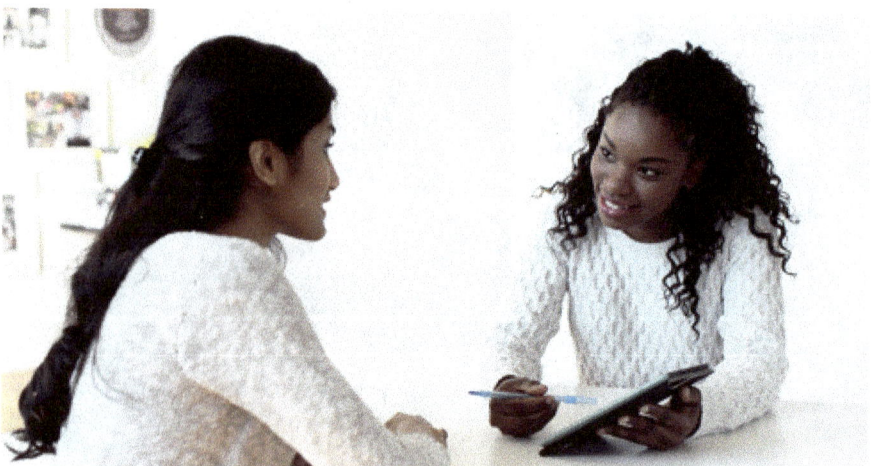

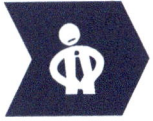

If you lock your hands behind your neck or head this indicates arrogance.

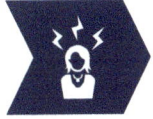

If you point with your finger or you are wagging it in front of them this is aggression.

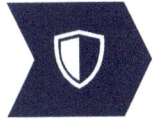

When you cross your arms, you are defensive.

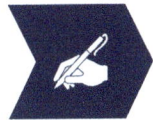

When you play with your pen, you are bored.

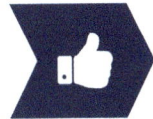

When you twiddle your thumbs, you are nervous.

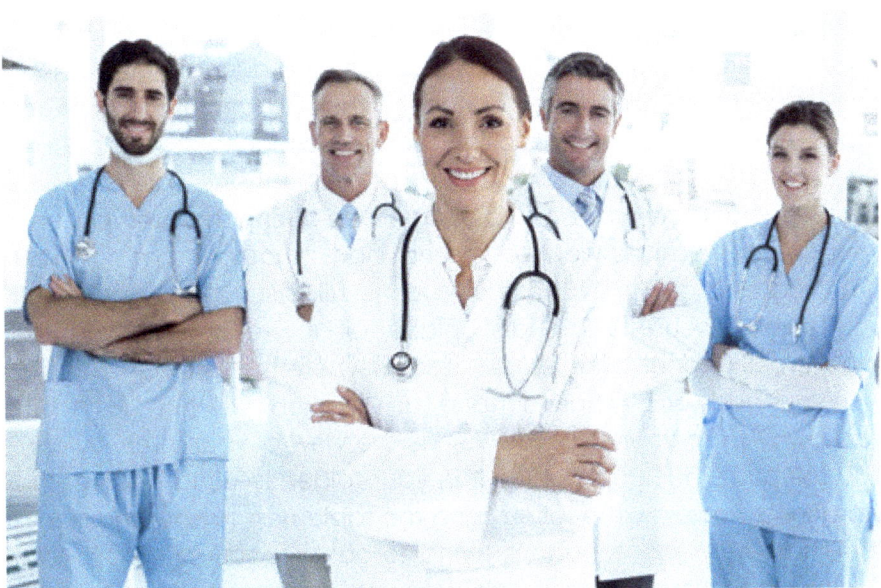

4.7 Distractions- Phones

With the increasing desire, supply and demand of new technology becoming integrated into our lives at a faster and more frequent pace, it seems that people are getting progressively kitted out with gadgets and gizmos, always seeking for the latest fashion, new attire, new benefits and features. We're not in the year 2100 yet so for now you do not need to arrive at the interview completely plastered in technology unless it is something necessary of course. These days, the two most common items are the mobile/cell phone and the smart watch. You need to show the interview panel sitting across the table that you are self-organised, proactive and that you think on your feet. If you attend the interview with technology over half your body weight then you have greater chances for distractions to occur, both for the interviewers and yourself. If you have a mobile phone, please switch it off or put it on silent mode. It is very impolite for your phone to ring when you are in an interview. Otherwise as a result you may receive a sarcastic comment from one of the panel members such as "Oh, could you tell them that I am not available to answer right now as I am busy conducting an interview?". Not a good start, and so it begins. "I'm sorry, where is a safe place to put it so as to not interrupt or disturb the interview?" does not sound like a good ice-breaker does it? If it ever does sound during the interview, you can start by immediately cancelling the call, switching it on silent mode, apologising and proposing for it to be placed in your pocket, bag or folder. The pocket is the most convenient and easy place to use. But what if it is on silent/vibrating mode during the interview and your friends/relatives want to find out how it has gone or how you are progressing? Surely these vibrations will disturb you and derail your trail of thoughts. The ideal place for any technology such as mobile/cell phones to be stored is somewhere that is not in contact with your body or any hard surface (as vibrations will then be heard) and away from your view (as well as the view of your interviewers). You therefore decide to place it in your folder so as to not feel the vibrations. However, the folder is on the table next to you and again the same story, somebody is trying to contact you to review your position and your success. This time the phone is on silent mode but now the vibrations are resonating the whole table. Everybody is aware of it and the whole interview is interrupted. A fact like that can very easily make the interviewers stop the process and keep the interview short. This is not a good thing if at that time you had gained momentum and you have them cornered in a very interesting topic which had given you extra points. All these are now potentially completely lost by somebody who was rightfully anxious about you because they care about you. It is not the fault of the caller. They want to learn of your progress. The fault is in fact all yours who has carelessly allowed your phone to ring by failing to prepare and failing to think of all possible hurdles. That is why I stated previously that it would be better to keep the folder next to your seat. Even if the phone vibrates it is not going to disturb you or the panel. Now that you have planned prior to the interview, you have all the time to freely and calmly continue your progress with no distractions. Do not leave a fact of chance to ruin you. It is much better though for a phone to be switched off and you have peace in mind.

4.8 Negative Influences & Impacts- Chewing Gum

When you are answering the questions keep on smiling and looking at them straight in the eyes. You know, smiling is not a permanent frozen position of your mouth and face, trying to imitate Mona Lisa. Smiling is also a feeling and this can very easily be seen in the eyes, easier than you think. The eyes can smile while the mouth talks. Only after the sentence and talking have finished the smile returns to the mouth. Practise this at home, using all the available people, relatives, neighbours or friends as the members of the panel. With this practise you have the cognition to use the same technique with the interviewers. One common trick is to look yourself in the mirror and practise. This is the "mirroring" technique. Observe all your expressions and correct them. Originally, look at the person who made the question, but when answering keep looking at all of them. Eye contact is key. You need to build a rapport with them. As you can see, no matter how many times this has been stated previously, preparation is paramount and can eliminate your anxiety.

4.9 Voice Yourself

You must not see the interview as your examination from the institution, but rather as an experience. It is your chance to go on stage and promote yourself. It is your chance to "sing" along your own tunes. Please control the pitch of your voice and metaphorically, do not sing on Alto-Soprano when your voice is suited for Mezzo-Soprano. The voice will become distorted. Practise will teach you how to control yourself. Do not let the nerves get to your voice, the whole idea is nothing else than to say your story, that's it!

4.10 Stay Positive & Remember Your Core Values

You need to be honest, as you are nothing else other than yourself. When you tell your story, you do not mention your entire life story, family history or how many times you were told off by your mother (believe me, I have interviewed countless candidates and I have heard many of stories). All you need to do is arrive happy and prepared, answer their questions (no right or wrong, they just want to see if you will fit in their team, and if not then it does not matter, move onto the next one). Just mention how many and what good deeds you made in your life. Describe a scene (an important one) of your life, but avoid giving a lengthy play. This is exactly what the interview is about. Do not fear it, there truly is no need. It is simply a conversation, a friendly game. Just go to play in their playground and play well. Feel yourself as if you are in a team, your team, and you are going to compete in an away match. The grass of the stadium is the same, it's just grass! The differences are the facilities and the size of the stadium. You start from the second division and you are going to play in the first. So what! Go and enjoy the game. If you go with a liberated spirit, you will win. You will win because you will play without nerves. Release yourself, freedom and enjoyment are everything in life. This does not apply only to interviews. That is why when you come out of the room you will walk high and proud, smiling, and all because you enjoyed yourself. If you do this you win the spectators over. Did you know that the psychology of the panel is mixed? Did you think that they too may in fact feel nervous? Did you know that they too are also part players and part spectators in that team? So, try to win these spectators over, play an honest game with some good moments and sure, perhaps some bad moments, but do not be afraid to play. Sometimes you may think you played worse than you actually did. You may feel as if you did not win the game, but perhaps the commentators and spectators still enjoyed the match and may offer you a different league/division or even perhaps something more than you were actually expecting. Just continue to play. Keep your psychology high and come out smiling again, relaxed and happy. Who do you think will win at the end? You; only you. Even if you do not get what you wanted, perhaps you got something more valuable, the experience. Now, I said that you have to play a game which can impress the spectators. So do not think that you will be a winner by jumping into the stadium deliriously happy and coming out again jumping out of joy without any performance during the game. No, you will not. If so, you would probably be closer related to being the entertainer mascot that performs before and after in the intervals of the big game, whereby somebody else plays the serious game. This person, the big player, represents everybody else who applied for the same position as you did. Do not allow yourself to play the role of a clown.

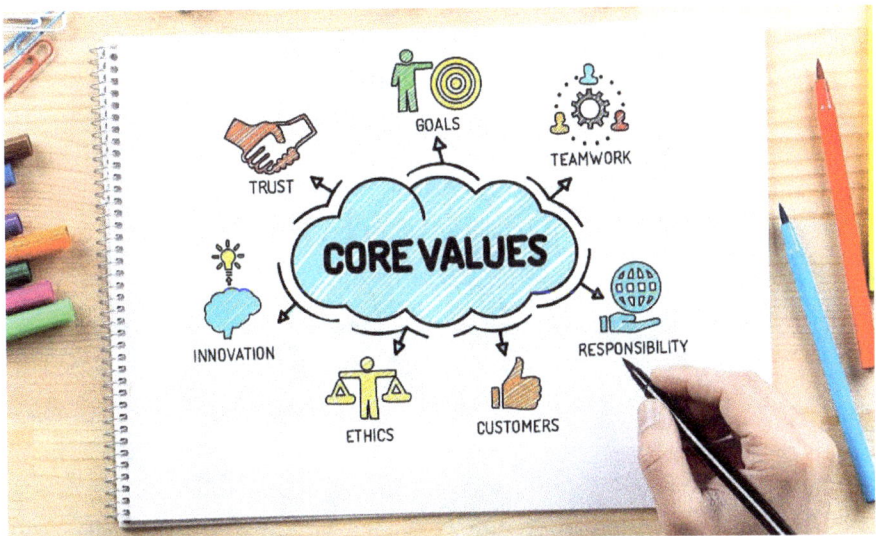

4.11 Endgame- The Finale

When the end of the interview is approaching and you have the feeling of this happening, try to summarise and promote your strengths. Now is the time. Show them with a conclusive summary that you are the person they are looking for and why you want to be part of their team. There are times however, whereby the interviewers are satisfied and stop the interview without a closing statement or much of a warning, thanking you for your presence and participation. Do not start summarising at that time, because this shows that you are out-of-sync and detached from the panel. You just thank them for the opportunity which they gave you and leave the room. As previously said, walk straight with a proud posture and a smile on your face. They may offer a handshake again. Do not deny this opportunity. Make sure that your hands are not sweating and shake their hands with your firm non crushing handshake, as mentioned before. If your hands are sweating you may be able to get away with giving them a subtle wipe on your trousers as you stand up for the handshake. Handshakes usually occur when both parties are stood up, so if a panel member stands to shake your hand please ensure you do too. Do not stay seated and shake their hand while seated. This is the continuation of the communication with them and part of the rapport that both parties have created. Additionally, shaking of the hands at the end is sometimes a very good sign. If you feel that you performed well and they offer their hand to you, it may seem like they closed the deal with you. Again, if no hand shake is offered, or the size of the table is too big, you should address them with a polite gesture of your head as you previously did when you came into the room. Proceed by calmly walking out while thanking them for the opportunity.

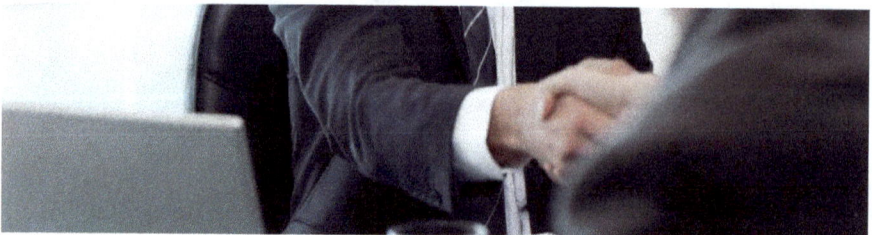

4.12 And Breathe

Now you are out of the stuffy interview room and into the clean air. Believe me the interview may have ended, but the observations of yourself are still continuing. Firstly, you need to observe yourself. If you come out, not feeling numb but instead you feel fine as if nothing happened, then this indicates that you were relaxed in the room, which is positive.

Furthermore, as soon as you are out, people such as family, friends or other candidates may surround you to learn how things went or may ask the context of the questions. It is good to tell them, express your feelings and get it off your chest because this way you can reflect back upon what the interview was like. Now with clear mind you can review the process and clarify the situation within your mind. You may even not remember all the details. It is normal if you even feel a little blank. Please note you do not have to say everything either if you do not want to. Do not feel forced to say anything. You need to understand the experience yourself firstly before letting others know about it.

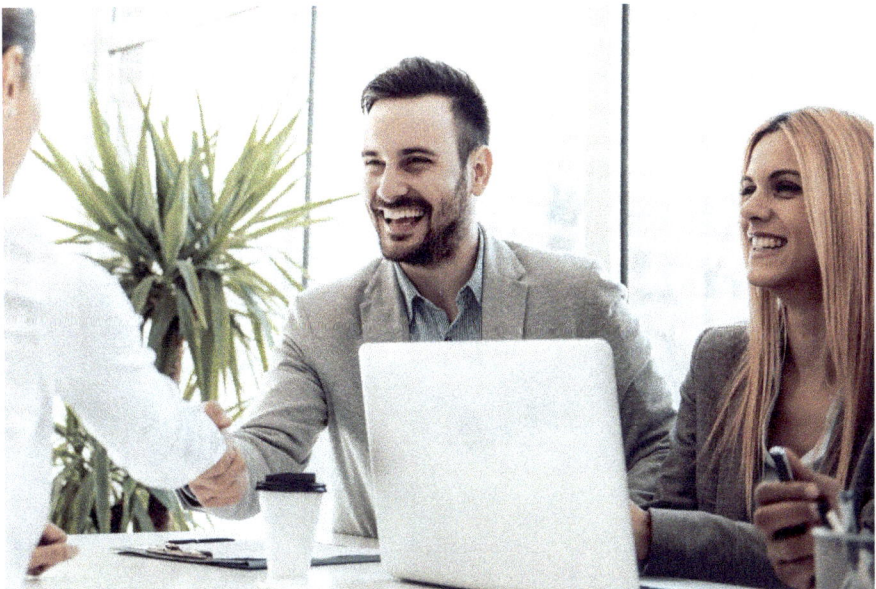

4.13 Tips

Here is some advice, a small trick to help you now. Usually for the sake of having a baseline for comparison, the interviewers ask the same or similar themed questions. It is true and obvious that they receive different answers from every individual candidate in front of them, however, sometimes for the clarification of the answer they may explore with further additional questions. The great news though is that the initial questions that each of them does is possibly common and generic to every candidate. As I said they may not be the exact ones but of a similar theme. Can you now read between the lines? If another candidate comes out and you are not the next, you can approach this person and learn the pattern of the questions. You can follow the theme as well as the categories of questions therefore becoming better prepared, and stronger. You can utilise this when you can, however also be wary of other candidates trying to throw you off. That being said, in a lot of cases interview slots are organised in such a way those candidates will not encounter one another.

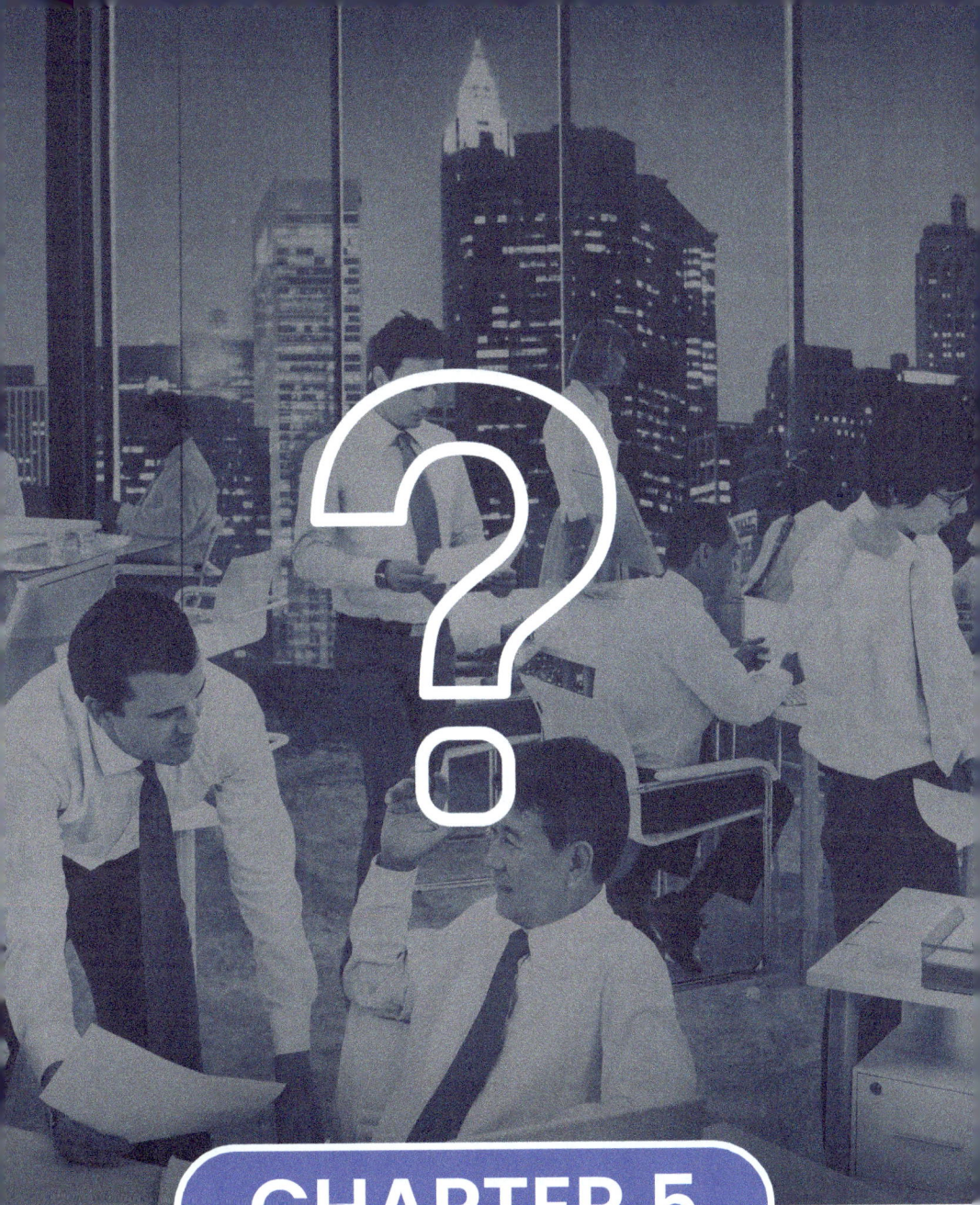

CHAPTER 5

FREQUENTLY ASKED QUESTIONS

In this part you will see some of the most common questions that are asked in an interview for Medicine. If you have been involved with any different interviews, you may find that some questions are common to all interviews from all industries around the world, however more focussed and geared towards Medicine. Please take the below descriptions and explanations as indication. You will need to spend some time yourself to explore the topics. Do not learn them off by heart. Use the following as momentum.

5.1 General Questions

1. Tell me about yourself / Can you talk me through your CV?

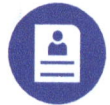

In such a question you have to expand your answers on your statement/CV. Do not forget that the statement/CV is a summary of your life and now you have the opportunity to enter the details. It is time for you to sell yourself, big time. This is an open question which is gives you every chance to expand upon yourself but also for the panel to check the statement's integrity and honesty. Be professional though and do not go through personal emotions. Open yourself but do not expose yourself. You are not under the spotlight of the interrogation party neither you are lying on your psychotherapist's couch.

2. Why do you want to become a doctor/nurse/health professional?

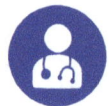

Speak about the influence which made you decide to follow the profession. Speak about your understanding of Medicine and talk through the potential strengths that you have in relation to the demands which medicine places upon medical professionals. You already analysed this in previous chapter. Think about how and which way you could overcome all these difficulties. Mention your weaknesses as well, describing how you could overcome them and turn them into strengths. Do not stay at the weaknesses without mentioning the potential solution or stating how you intend to resolve them. Describe how you will use these to develop, how you will battle them out of your system. You have to show that you are positive but human. This has to be evident at all times. If you do not mention strengths and weaknesses the interviewers will ask you about them anyway at some stage, so do it before them. There is a possibility that they will pin point one of the strengths and/or one of the weaknesses, so be prepared. Try to have a more in-depth analysis of everything you mention to them in case you need the answer when they ask you.

3. What is your greatest achievement?

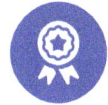

Here you have to mention something that you are proud of and how this affected you, why this was important to you and how it made you feel. This is part of you and may not have any relation with Medicine. This is potentially a personal question so technically there is no wrong answer, however the interviewers will try to pick out behaviour, characteristics and sense of achievement that they find relatable to their team. You must be able to share experiences and work towards common goals. This question shows the panel the ability that you have to reflect and how you can learn from it. If this is in sport for example, you can talk about teamwork and commitment. You can discuss how this will affect your career in Medicine. Conversely, this question can easily be asked on the negative side by asking to describe your greatest failure. Be prepared and show how you have learned from the experience. This is reflection.

4. How do you describe yourself?

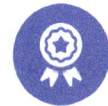

Another reflective question. You need to analyse yourself. It is nothing else than a combination of the previous questions. You need to show your motivation and how this is represented in your CV. Describe the positive way that you approach problems and how you could solve the challenges. Additionally, you will need to reflect towards your examples which will include your achievements. You need to show that you are a team player and are able to provide a set example. Motivation and initiative are almost synonyms, so prepare yourself accordingly. Mention the reasons and the ways that stimulate your motivation. Talk about your creativity, your ability to build bridges and work in teams.

5. How do you act/perform under pressure/stress?

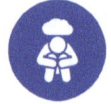

Here you need to indicate the difference which exists between the meaning of the word pressure and stress. Pressure is not stressful at all times. Too much pressure may be stressful and believe it or not even not enough pressure may be equally so. Prepare yourself and show how pressure sometimes acts in a positive way and stress in a negative way. Discuss how you can work happily under pressure but how stress can be destructive. Show how you have the ability to change stress to pressure by channelling it towards your work performance and talk about your robust inner world. Demonstrate how you communicate under pressure and you seek help from more experienced people in these difficult times. This is usually a question they will get the answer to without you realising. After all, you are supposedly in a "stressful" situation right now during the interview, so keep your cool and think about everything that was previously discussed above.

6. Can you describe the ideal person for the post/job?

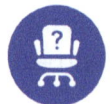

Again, this is an open question. Do not be afraid because it looks personal. This is about the strength that a doctor has to have, and in parallelism as you are describing the characteristics of a good doctor, you just say about yours. Remember the qualities a doctor has to have. So, sell yourself.

7. What is your experience in Medicine to date?

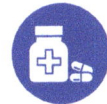

With this open question you go back to your CV and pick the experiences that you had when you were placed as an attachment into the different hospitals or practices. As you are aware, work experience plays a major part in you being accepted for an interview into the School of Medicine, so it is vital for you to sell yourself in this experience. Never talk about bad experiences or people in a negative way. If ever asked specifically about negative experiences you need to show them how you resolved the issues in a professional manner. Show them how you handled the situation positively, and what you learnt from it.

8. Why do you believe that you can achieve this and be successful in Medicine? What makes you think you will be a successful/ good medical professional/Doctor later on in your career/life?

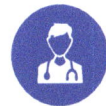

Talk about your motivation, your ability to work in a team, starting from your vision and your goals. Show how determined you are to achieve it all, as your fulfilment of the qualities of a good doctor.

9. What do you think a doctor can do, except the treatment of patients?

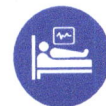

All this is based on your background preparation. Talk about research and future scientific achievements or even education, managerial positions in health schemes and services. Prepare for this by doing research into the function of the National Health Service (NI IS in the U.K.) and public services.

10. If you were in our position what would you ask yourself?

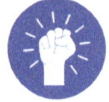

Tricky? Certainly not. Base this question on your strengths and develop the question. Justify the question and then answer it for yourself, while increasing the positive parts of yourself.

11. After reading the University information pack, what appealed to you and what made you follow this course?

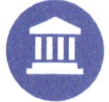

Here it is, your research and how all the information you received during the open day and from the pack now interconnects with your personal statement and previous experiences. Describe how, in your opinion, all this has influenced you in the way that you applied for this University. You can talk about other packs which you have researched and compare them with the present. Be careful not to mention the names of the other institutions. It is not necessary. If, in case you are directly questioned "which packs are they?", you openly suggest that you would prefer not to mention. This will be appreciated as well as respected as you hold back the privacy.

12. Do you think there are any advantages or disadvantages when you study Medicine?

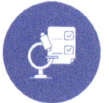

This is another open question, stressing on your personal abilities and reflection as well as the way that you will develop within Medicine. Think about the qualities of a doctor. They may question you since they want to explore to what degree your interest in Medicine resonates and how far you went on your research. They may ask you about Hippocrates, the father of Medicine; the medical achievements in the recent years and your opinion about them; if you read any medical papers which helped you to make up your mind on a career path; any particular event which turned you towards Medicine (this could be a book, a film, a scientific paper or even an article in the local newspapers, but also a life event).

13. They may ask you questions about the redistribution of wealth, as "Do you think it is right for countries to spend copious amounts of money for the Olympic Games every four years (or build upon/innovate technology for weapons/warfare, or send people into space)? Is money well spent? If now you had the same amount of money, how would you spend it?".

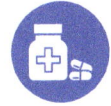

Here you should have a plan for re-distribution of the wealth and you need to justify your answers. Do not forget you need multiple answers here, as there are multiple questions.

14. They may ask you about your hobbies.

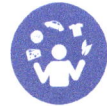

You may ask; Hobbies, why are they so important? Hobbies can show others part of your personality, so think about them and reflect finding the positives and the negatives. Concentrate on promoting the positives. They may question you about a theoretical role of you in a team and how this would work/change if you were to gradually be involved at different levels in the team. A correlation may also be made between your interests in a team (e.g. football) and how you believe this would look like if represented in the National Health Service (NHS in the U.K.). In these cases, you should base yourself upon your research in that the way the NHS works and how you need to support it with your actions.

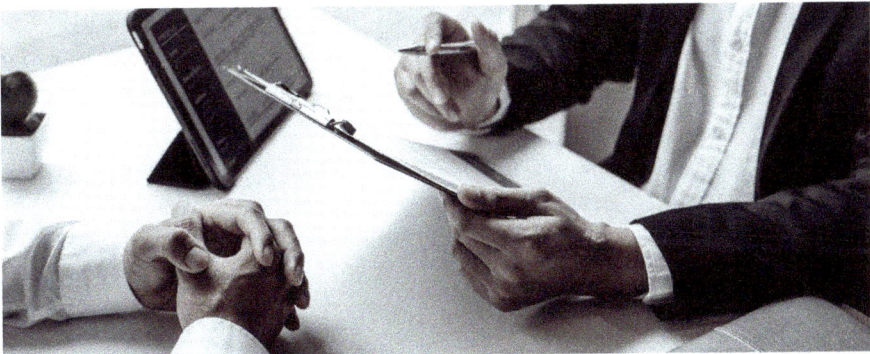

5.2 Additional Queries

Further questions to demonstrate your understanding of the NHS, the problems it faces, the limitations which exist or benefits that we as professionals may have, can also be asked. They may ask your opinion about:

The waiting lists

Money expenditure

Lack of funding

How managers and politicians influence the work of doctors and health workers.

You can find all these answers as you research into the NHS via websites and newspapers, but also ask and discuss with the professionals currently experiencing all the above during your work experiences/attachments. Learn and think about the effect that the press/media has in general on the doctor-patient relation and how this can be manipulated by the political powers. Your position has to be based on these publications, but do not express any political views. AVOID POLITICS. They may ask you about the relationship between science and medicine, or your opinion about the ethics of new developments in medicine, such as cloning, animal experiments and animal rights, how these can be conducted in a humane way or if they are even necessary. They will ask these questions in order to see if you are aware of developments in the field and alert of medical research. This will show them that you understand the direction of the profession and where it is heading. They may wish to discuss your volunteer work and the reasons which drove you to undertake this task. This way they will explore the obscured corners of your personality.

5.3 The Close- Be Impactful, Stay Professional & Ethical

I hope that all these tips and sample questions within these guidance notes can holistically stimulate your imagination to aid the creation of all the necessary parts for a sound foundation, helping you piece together and easily create the puzzle that opens the gates for you to follow Medicine in a limitless and effective manner.

One more point, after your interview when you leave, if you have the opportunity try to write a letter to the University/Institution/Organisation thanking them for the opportunity they gave you to experience an interview with them, then please do so. Please be mindful of this. This should be done despite and regardless of the resulting outcomes.

5.4 The Inspirational Bit- It has been Emotional

Finally, I wish you the very best of luck. Stay focused on your goals and satisfy your dreams, which is to serve your patients. This can be achieved through your clinical skills, but also through teaching and mentoring where you can provide the future generations of doctors with a solid grounding. Become a role model to these juniors. Show them how to do things ethically, professionally, properly and well. Pass down your experiences, the good and bad. Give them your knowledge and teach them how to treat patients the way you would want to be treated, because one day they will be the ones that treat you.

Lastly to conclude, you may wish to explore new frontiers in the fields of further research for the betterment of our great science and systems but mainly for the improvement of services of our patients. You can even involve yourself with public health as well as the management of the health services and systems. No matter your choice, whether it be management, practitioner, surgeon, researcher and so on, you will find out that the greatest gift and most fulfilling payback that you will receive during your career is nothing else than the smile of a patient and/or their loved ones, the heart-warming handshake deeply and wholeheartedly thanking you for your services, the cheers as an announcement gets made about a major scientific breakthrough. Live for these moments, never forget them and make it so they are frequent. Yes, you will have unhappy people and you will make mistakes, after all you are only a human being, but even these moments will be your enlightenment, helping you understand and make progress. These trying times will move you forwards. Seek the job satisfaction and the thing you will remember the most will be that smile, those achievements. Medicine is based on the existence of the human interest, the pursue of a better, more comfortable life for the sick. It is founded on the altruism of the doctor, the other health workers and on the progression of the science, with all the possible ethical means that we implement now. We need to apply the technology of today, remember the techniques and technology of yesterday and plan to discover the technology of tomorrow. If you choose to be involved with Medicine (and I wish you to do so), try to involve yourselves and your clinical duties with patient management, whatever this may be. Please serve Medicine honourably and be proud of it. GOOD LUCK!

In the next chapter you will find some examples of statements which you can read for your benefit as previously mentioned.

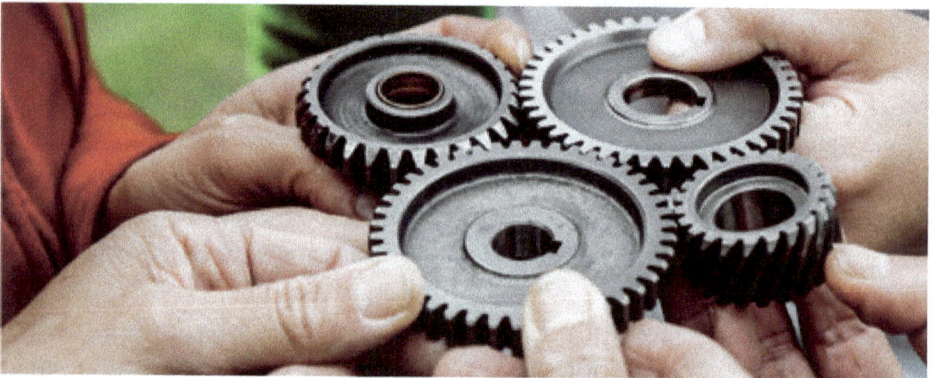

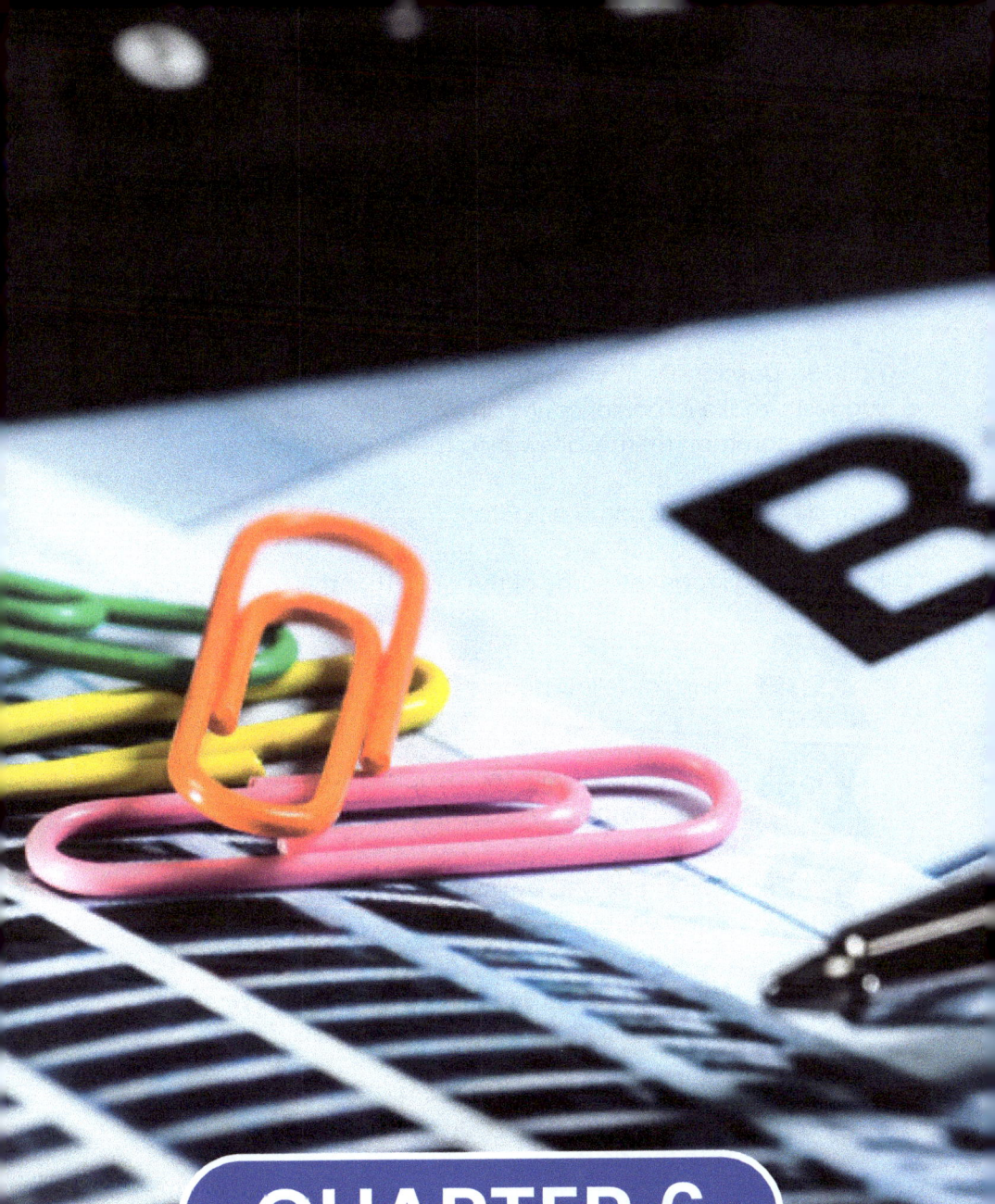

CHAPTER 6

APPENDIX

In this chapter you will be exposed to some summarised, fictional and general Personal Statement ideas so that you can have a rough guideline (or a gentle nudge in the good direction) on what different types of information you should include in your own, whilst keeping in mind how the stories flow.

Tips? Be passionate in your stories/descriptions, and as the name suggests, make it "personal". As an example, all the below ideas will follow a common theme; answering the main question:

"Why do I want to become a Doctor?"

The following ideas are some of the ways that this is answered:

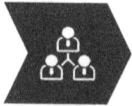

Help my fellow people (I like to physically help lives)

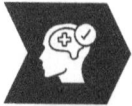

Be in contact with the people (I like to mentally help lives, psychology & psychiatry)

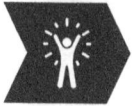

Self-influenced by illness in the family (personal experiences)

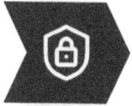

The NHS is the world's fifth largest employer which would offer security (job & financial security)

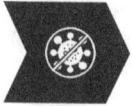

Eliminate diseases (reduce poverty, old/past illnesses, bring poor parts of the world up to date with the developed world)

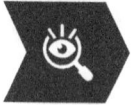

Find new cures (future technology & research)

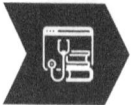

I am good at the modules/subjects that are required to enter a Medical course at University

Now let's go into a little more detail for each of the above.

6.1 Idea 1- Help my Fellow People

The first thought that crosses my mind is that I need to attend to and care about people who are unable to care for themselves. These are people in need, people in pain and despair. You can see by the way these people look at you as a fellow person, that their eyes are full of questions about their condition. Whether they are worried for themselves or their loved ones whose systems are not working well, they are desperate to solve these problems of suffering. To see their smile and receive their gratitude after the treatment would make me feel full of love and joy. Knowing that you have provided hope that they can now move their lives forward is the greatest and purest fulfilment that I believe in. These priceless feelings would make me smile both inside and out. Devoting my life to a profession that minimises or even eliminates the need for people to be pushing themselves to limits whilst going to great lengths in order to cope with illnesses that have no easy cures would be life's greatest accomplishment. I believe with my support they can achieve what they desire and live a dignified life. The more people that are treated the greater the feeling, especially when you get to experience people standing proudly, steady and straight when previously they may have been bedbound. I would have been part of the team that made this happen and allow them to leap over their previous difficulties as well as assist and coach them through the dire straits. I have a passion for listening to and helping people so as to stop that lonely feeling one gets in the contact of diseases, reassuring them that they have a shoulder to lean on and a bond to support them throughout their lives when in difficulty. I want to be able to help people live a life of good quality and these are the reasons that drive me to become a doctor.

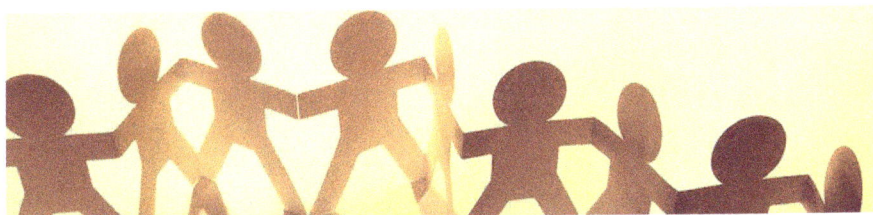

6.2 Idea 2- Be in Contact with the People

As a person I like being in contact with people and have always welcomed people who seek help. I use my good listening skills to engage with their problems and find possible solutions using my experiences and knowledge. I have found myself in many situations where I listen to people's problems and find it both fascinating and rewarding when I involve myself to overcome one's difficulties. I am not afraid or uncomfortable being close to people in times of difficulty to discuss the details of how they can get through the dire straits that they walk. Humans are programmed to communicate between themselves and I feel to be an effective communicator. Using this skill, I can enable people to make contact and possibly offload their bad or conflicted feelings or else thoughts, allowing them to better understand their situation from all perspectives in order to get deeper into the root causes, thus closer to finding a solution. Being the person I am, I feel that I give great help to my fellow humans. I love the potential and possibility of opening a door whereby problems are on the other side in need of confrontation, liaising with patients where I am able to ease their confidence towards comfort and offer my support without asking for payment in return. The satisfaction of knowing that I have greatly impacted and positively influenced someone's life in addition to seeing them walk back out the same door they once walked in earlier, with fewer problems while metaphorically opening another door in front of them is more than enough of a reimbursement for me. I strive to make people feel the presence of my company so that they feel free, comfortable and protected in a respectful, professional and confidential environment. People need to be safe at all times but when they are in vulnerable, sensitive or unstable situations, this need of safety must be emphasised. As being in contact with people is a passion, I offer myself to their services for their own wellbeing. Initially, I never thought that communication alone was enough to initiate a person's treatment but now I am convinced that this is the beginning of everything. Communication is the key route in solving any trouble. As people, we appreciate, grow to like and learn to open up when we show care to one another. Communication through positive, efficient and effective ways is what is needed. Humour can also pave the way to aid in opening up, breaking the ice and allowing them even just for a moment to forget everything that they came in for. Relief is what they are asking for. This applies to both patients and their families, and by having this ability I believe I will become a successful doctor, spreading my knowledge so people can better self-deal with issues.

6.3 Idea 3- Self-Influenced by Illness in the Family

It was from a young age that I decided to become a doctor as I was involved in difficult personal experiences. My Grandmother who I loved a lot, was involved in an accident which resulted in her being admitted to the local hospital where I remember her being in the Accident & Emergency Department. All the doctors and nurses were attending to and surrounding her while she was lying on the trolley. We were asked to patiently stay in a separate area where I then saw them wheeling her to other areas for X-Rays and further investigations. Finally, she was admitted to the ward where again she had great attention, followed by the operating theatre where they fixed the broken bones before returning her back to the ward. My Grandmother had daily care where her needs were attended to for the entirety of three weeks before being safely discharged from the hospital, returning home. She would walk in small distances with walking aids and went back and forth to the hospital to be seen by the doctors where finally, six months following the accident she was fully discharged. This whole "roller-coaster adventure" in my family marked my mind during my childhood and I felt full of admiration for the people who cared so much for my Grandmother as if she were their family. My mind was now engraved. I could not believe how an injured, crippled person, unable to move due to being very sick and in a lot of pain with damaged bones and multiple wounds, once again became an active person, someone now able to walk and even dance (my Grandmother loved to dance). She had no more pain; she was happy once again. With the help, perseverance and integrity of the doctors and nurses, this would not have been possible. Her scarred face from the pain was now enlightened with smiles of joy. This was the turning moment in which I decided to become a doctor as I too wanted to be someone who can bring so much relief, so much joy to a people and their families alike as they did for me by caring for, mending and comforting the lives of others.

6.4 Idea 4- The NHS is the World's Fifth Largest Employer

In the present financial climate, there is great insecurity for the future of a young person. The majority of the employers live in an environment which is variable. There is a possibility that somebody spends all their years studying in University only to then discover that they are unable to find work, and even if they are lucky to be employed, it is sometimes difficult to retain the employment as there is a chance for the company of employment to become bankrupt or make the employee redundant due to ever-changing times, technology and roles. So, the key is to make a choice at the beginning, a forecasted projection to find an organisation with life-long employment that offers enough security for a stable life and the possibility to raise a stable family. Checking the international market and the international companies with kudos, I discovered that the NHS is the fifth largest international employer with the most employees, so I searched further. The NHS was established immediately after the Second World War to protect all citizens of Britain and give them the equal opportunity for a safe and healthy life. It was at a time of necessity that everybody was united under this idea as this was necessary for the people who suffered a lot following this blood thirsty war. All had embraced this idea of a Welsh politician and now the NHS has grown to an organisation with great numbers of employees, continuing to resonate the same motto for years to come, "Equal opportunity to health for everyone". The idea of helping all by the few health workers is great, it is empowering and captivating. Simultaneously, the employment is stable and the future more secure than in any other industry, therefore this is a very easy choice for me. As I believe in strength comes through unity, I found the NHS compelling due to its backbone nature for a national system as well as the desire to carry out my passion of aiding people. Combining stability with satisfaction of an honourable profession that works towards the betterment and improvement of mankind is why I would like to become a doctor! What more could somebody want for their life?

6.5 Idea 5- Eliminate Diseases

During my early years in the school, I was fascinated by the different documentaries on the television where they would describe different civilisations of the many countries. I noticed that some countries were very poor and had no facilities when compared to my own. Growing up, this would constantly be on my mind and I would feel very sorry about the situations some countries have to deal with when so much to resolve these issues already exist, so this inspired, pushed and drove me towards finding out more. My goal has always been to find ways to which I can help these people in need by looking into the different reasons as to why issues were apparent. One of the many reasons that I found was also possibly the most important part of their lives, the absence of good health. These are people who either have no clean water, houses with no welfare facilities or no houses at all, lack of drainage systems but mainly people without education on how to recognise the dangerous and threatening

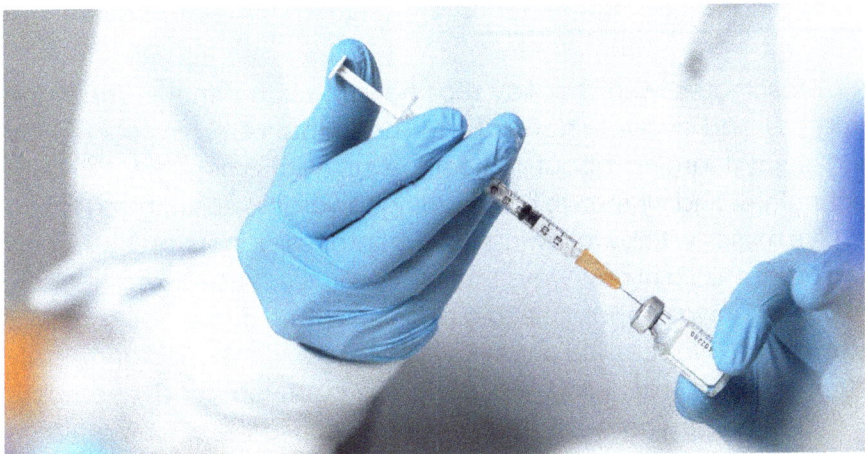

conditions. Further into my search I found that there are people who are exposed to the elements of nature. I noticed that these people were bombarded by diseases that were eliminated in my country a long time ago. The names of Tuberculosis, Poliomyelitis, Cholera and Leprosy were very common diseases amongst them. However, at the present time all these diseases have been eliminated in the civilised world due to vaccination programmes or improved hygiene (education) whereas these diseases still exist in the third world. I decided I would like to become a doctor in order to go to these deprived areas and places because I wanted to be involved with something that matters, something that can make a change and be part of the teams that help these people acquire an improved quality of life. Facilitating their education was a great personal desire, to improve their status and knowledge thus increasing their life expectancy without decreasing the pleasure they had by living in these remote paradise places. They needed to be able to live a better quality of life but without destroying their environment. The more I found out the more I wanted to help and turn these places into self-sufficient systems, in order to replicate the rest of the world, turning common diseases into whispers of the past. I wanted to assist them with achieving this requirement while eliminating the danger and suffering that they experienced because of diseases that are already extinct in our world.

5.2 Idea 6- Find New Cure

I am fascinated with the way that new developments in medicine progress and evolve. I have always been interested in technology and enjoy learning about it. Keeping up with where we are with technology and where we are heading towards is something I like to involve myself with by following documentaries, papers, articles, news and other media of new ways that we can investigate diseases. Many years ago, it was impossible to diagnose something unless a clinical examination was carried out. X-Rays were then developed and slowly introduced into medicine. Watching this captivating advancement unfold over the years, I started to get a real sense of how limitless progress can be. Medicine has developed and continues to do so in such a rate that you cannot think or believe that almost 25 years ago there were investigation styles unknown to us which current medical staff would have never experienced. To see for example, if somebody's knee had a damaged cartilage there would be no other ways apart from either having to open it, or to use special X-Rays to image it and prove that something was wrong. These X-Rays carried the inherent high risk of false positive or false negative results. Now, through the development of the Magnetic Resonance Imaging (MRI) scans we have the ability, with a 95% success, to diagnose soft tissue injuries that were previously not possible to diagnose in such a high rate without the need of operational and surgical intervention. The advances made in molecular medicine and genetic science now give us, for the first time, the opportunity not only to diagnose the common diseases that are distressing us but to also gain indication of ways to even cure members of the community that are yet to become ill (e.g. heart disease, diabetes etc.). The thoughts of eliminating congenital diseases by studying people's DNA and that one day we may have the complete understanding to cure cancer is so inspiring. I would like to be an involved member of such a team, to participate in a great cause and work towards acquiring the much-sought in-depth knowledge and understanding that will help pave the way towards cures of diseases. This strong and fulfilling feeling is the reason why I would like to become a doctor!

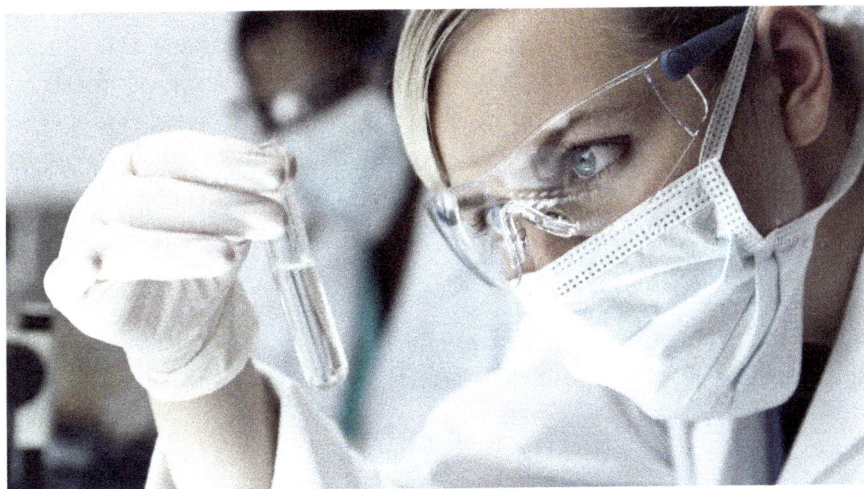

6.7 Idea 7– I am good at the modules/subjects that are required to enter a Medical course at University

Throughout my life I studied hard with one goal in mind, my ambition was to go to University. The decision to choose a course was very difficult as I had to marry passion with life-fulfilment. Knowing I had to make an important decision and resolve this concern by coming out of the confused condition, I started to identify which lessons/topics I was performing the best in and which desires I possessed for my life. As soon as I made this active decision, things became very clear to me. I had therefore found a tool I could use which then guided me to make a decision. As I believe topic subjects required for course entry into university represent the mentality, logicality and methodology needed to progress in addition to the way courses are taught, I used the list of subjects I performed well in to guide me to a course I would enjoy and flourish in. My mentality needed to match the mentality of the future education within the course. I found that over the years Mathematics, Physics, Chemistry & Biology, were strong subjects of mine. Additionally, language subjects such as English & French were positive. Following further investigation and analysis with grading and more, it was apparent that Biology was the strongest subject, followed by the rest of the Sciences as Physics and Chemistry. Some of the modules within Mathematics indicated strength however some parts of Mathematics I was not so strong, although using mathematical tools in Physics suggested that I could merge the subjects and solve complex problems. Finally, the language subjects such as English were sufficient enough to prove cognitive skills. Having thrown all this into the search of a course, I found that one of these courses that met my criteria was Medicine. Combining this with my love for improving and helping mankind this was the time I thought about the positive values that I would have in my life (satisfaction and fulfilment) if I followed this profession, and suddenly I fell in love with it. I decided I would be a doctor!

Other general examples of some statements based on how potential applicants should write and express themselves can be seen below.

You may for example have had previous undergraduate degrees or went through an observation program, thus the ideas/examples below have been tailored to cover these aspects too. Personal experiences on extracurricular activities also play a significant role in student selection for some Universities/Institutions/Organisations, therefore please take your time to describe these too. Nothing is more important than the rest you write about, everything is as important as the rest.

6.8 Example 1

Ever since I was young, I had a love for life and understood how precious it is. I cared for all flora and fauna, and whatever it was, I believed in preserving it. Throughout my life, I have always had an interest in science, especially biology as it can lead to many positive outcomes. Although I found biology to be my strongest and most enjoyable subject, I still found modules within it challenging and difficult to understand at first when compared to other modules, however I was determined and I endeavoured to achieve a level of understanding that lead to me teaching fellow peers out of class. I am a keen learner and would be delighted for an opportunity to expand my knowledge and skills by attending this course. The part that intrigued and drew me towards this fascinating subject was the complex, intricate detail nature has made to overcome age old problems, constantly changing and evolving to perfect what is otherwise a wonder. This led to rapidly gaining great interests in general medicine (e.g. veterinary and forensic) as well as how treatments are applied with paramedical and pharmacology sciences which resultod in my early decision to have a career in medicine.

Biology was one of my favourite modules and although it was difficult, it enabled me to closely study the anatomy of the human body. Since it was clear this was a passion of mine, I wanted to act on it, put it to good use and utilise my enthusiastic drive towards medical science while working with people in an ever-changing field that is critical to the world. Once I began the studies I never looked back. I have been involved with many projects and have gained high marks for my reports, however this was not always the case. Writing reports can become a bit of an art and is something I have learnt over the years with each report increasing my skills. This improvement in myself made me yearn for helping others with similar situations, therefore I ran a study club whereby I would aid in teaching how to research, read, write, present verbally, communicate, plan, time manage and improve overall comprehensive and literacy skills of students so they can have the chance to achieve what they desire. A lot of young students that attended would have dyslexia but a lot would also just want to be the best version of themselves. There were so many indirect benefits by holding these classes in which we all constantly learnt, even myself as the older year mentor, such as teamwork, and many went on to become friends through these classes. Regarding myself, I learnt how to take initiatives and accept responsibility through these classes. I did not have anything like this available to me in those years and saw it as a weakness as well as an opportunity for the school to develop further since I knew how difficult it could be to go through educational times like I did. I also found the psychology interesting of how the perception of younger adults was compared to students that did not need as much help as others. It was an eye-opening experience seeing these students help each other, the ones in greater need, somewhat becoming a self-sufficient class to such an extent that I took a step back to allow others to rise up and host the classes as we are species that wants to survive by science, improvements and advancement.

During my educational period I wanted to pursue more in order to construct real expectations of the path I chose. I therefore looked to gain experience first-hand from professionals by shadowing doctors, nurses and other medical staff in a General Hospital. I wanted to spend time with them in order to get a real sense of the medical life. The experience would consist of understanding the politics, seeing the pressure inflicted on staff during clinical sessions, observing the on-calls, ward rounds and learning about the different facilities (and when to use them). The path I wanted to take was yet to be clearly decided within the medical field, but I at least knew I preferred as well as enjoyed a lot more, the structural and systematic side of the human anatomy hence I drew my attention to surgery of various departments such as rheumatology, cardiology, orthopaedics and trauma. I wanted to get a feel of how things are done day to day as well as have a small taster of how things are managed in a totally different setting, unknown situation and environment as understood to be the nature of emergency situations whereby you need to decisively. After experiencing this vast insight of the medical life, it was clear to me that communication was crucial in reaching a conclusive diagnosis and in acting upon time limited situations with a swift but precisely calculated manner in order to achieve quality results. Within communication lies teamwork, whereby I saw much of first-hand. You could tell staff had built such trustworthy, synchronised and strong teams that there were cases when entire procedures were understood by few words. Everyone was so in-tune with each other and their environment that the operations that took place were smooth like an art. I learnt a lot during the days in theatre and enjoyed experiencing these instances to the extent that I began to want the same. My most recent work placement took place in a General Hospital whereby this confirmed and firmly set my decision

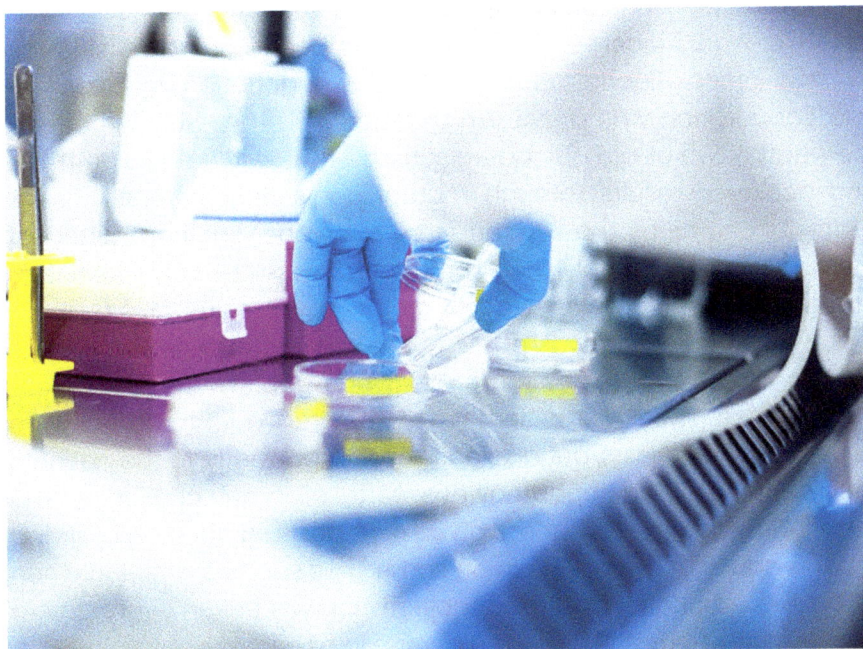

in stone to become a practitioner within medical science. There, I was exposed to visiting clinics, theatre surgeries that were performed by consultants, ward rounds and laboratory studies/testing. I found it fascinating how a collection of departments work together towards a common target, and how specialities of multiple teams produce each and every important piece to a complicated puzzle. Through these experiences I learnt how each surgery can have its own complexities and how important teamwork is. For example, when patients undergo Heart or Diabetic attacks multiple times during the operation for many reasons. I soon started to see and understand that each operation can comprise of numerous smaller operations that involve a vast amount of techniques as each is a unique surgery, having to overcome a series of hurdles whereby all avenues must be explored and all possible outcomes thought of, such as a hip replacement which incorporates bone grafts and metal plates to repair fractures, or patients with heart blockages within intensive care. Although my eyes were opened when observing doctors and consultants, I equally learnt just as much from talking to the patients themselves. This helped me piece together two sides of the story and allowed me to further grasp work from third year medical students under the supervision of the lead clinician. I have experienced a wide variety of work placements and each has been invaluable, such as the true place I learnt about teamwork, negotiation, involvement and cooperation was at a farm through voluntary work. Whatever the weather we all did our jobs, discussed the best ways to do them and achieved results through mutual goals and understandings. Team function was the key therefore everyone was committed to the vision. Following that, I then contributed myself to a special needs and mental health clinic/home whereby I saw a part of life that not many get to see. This was possibly the hardest experience to deal with as I saw that lives of some deprived people were so different to others like myself. Here I learnt how to listen, both to orders from nurses and specialists, but also and most importantly, to the patients themselves. I felt equipped however to take on any challenges the experience would throw at me given my nature, in addition to giving me the opportunity to hone in on some skills such as knowing when to be less emotional and more objective. I was driven every day to help and communicate with the people in need.

Looking ahead, I wish to be close to the people in order to help them understand their condition, ease their pain through comfort, and help them take the right steps forward to avoid further implications caused by illness through a guided journey. For this reason, I also volunteer and support a few charities such as the Heart Foundation in addition to children with disabilities such as autism by raising funds and helping students with skills improvement (e.g. reading, writing, computer literacy). It is a joy working with children and people with disabilities as it rewards everyone involved. I get great job satisfaction when I see how much happier they all get when interacting or getting involved with various activities. This past experience enlightened me on the vast range of disabilities and how, in reality, each one is very much unique. This resulted in acquiring communication skills and helped me to further connect with people which in turn opened up an even more fulfilling role. It is understood that these patients may show as well as inflict strains in families hence why I ensure time is taken to educate people as well as patients on how to become more self-sufficient and self-reliant. Moreover, I volunteered to take patients on trips to zoos and farms whereby they would feed goats and lamas, participate in nature walks and horse-riding. I mainly involved them with activities related to nature in order to connect easier with them and make them feel comfortable through these beneficial and therapeutic sessions. I found nature related activities worked best as nature runs deep inside us all. Similarly, further volunteer work was carried out with younger students to aid in resolving any issues or disagreements while offering them support and counselling if required as a school prefect and mediator. Issues may have consisted of exam fears, classmate relations, and general guidance for new students transitioning from primary to secondary school. This opportunity gave me the ability to ease people's lives, those who are in need and just wanted someone to express their feelings to. These experiences have been incredibly rewarding therefore I would like to pursue a career with lifetime satisfaction. For that reason, I want to study medicine, nursing, physiotherapy, psychology, the anatomy and the different effects pharmacology has on the body.

When I am not pursuing my passion of helping others, I am usually doing something to better myself by acquiring skills and learning how to do things such as DIY at home, gardening, or playing an instrument. I currently have a Grade 5 on guitar, and a Grade 3 on piano with music theory being Grade 6. I am currently working towards the higher grades on both instruments, as well as taking time to enjoy sport such as skiing, archery and horse-riding, but I sometimes combine the desire to help others with my love of sport and I participate in charity marathons. I feel as though being in the medical profession is something, like all things, that would need constant updating as well as learning and the best way to do this would be to get close to the people themselves and understand their issues first before attempting in find solutions. I try and do this every time I travel around the world by embedding myself into other people's culture.

Moving forward, in order to expand my experience further, I seek to carry out my next work experience at a General Practice whereby I look to increase my breadth of knowledge on how a Practice operates as well as the workings of a GP. This will bring me one step closer to the field, to the people in need and allow me to contribute to life preservation and distribution of knowledge for the benefit of others, making it a way of life and worthwhile career. Following these experiences and courses, I will be applying for an entry graduate level opportunity where I will be able to express my professionalism in terms of passion, reliability, hardworking nature, enthusiasm towards challenges, empathy and trustworthiness. Until then, I believe attending a university course such as this one will give me the right skills to move forward and put me in good stride to develop the strong foundation that a professional career such as this one needs.

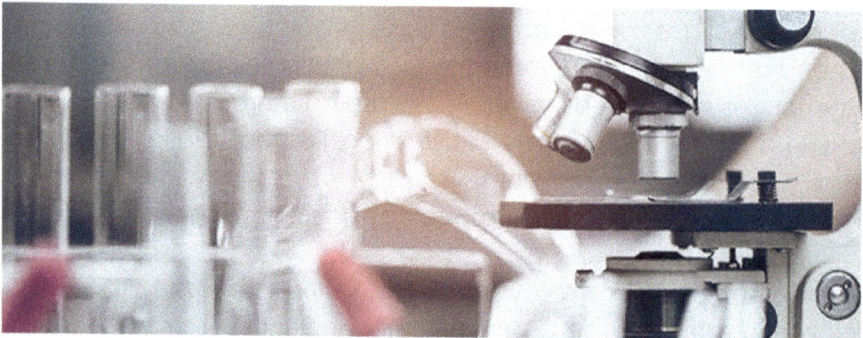

6.9 Example 2

Coming to the decision to follow a career in medicine was not always a childhood ambition of mine as many may think. Instead, I discovered that I enjoyed being there for people in need and as a matter of fact, all life. Certain life experiences have made it clearer to me that this is the path I should take and the life I should pursue. Experiences such as my love of life, voluntary work, helping children with special needs, travelling, improving lives of anyone I can and helping people with whatever they needed was something I first took for granted but later realised how this could be done on a grander scale as a career. I was always interested in health and getting the most out of our lives by being in the best position to do so. I enjoyed eating healthily, exercising regularly and guiding people to do the same. All this pushed me towards medicine, however I also enjoyed not only helping people biologically by caring for them, but also carrying out chores, constructing and creating physical solutions. I always had a creative side that needed satisfying through my "Engineering" mind but also craved the biological improvement of people's lives. By the end of high-school, I had decided I wanted to become an Orthopaedic Surgeon to satisfy my ambitions as it incorporated both health and mechanics. I was so fascinated and gravitated towards the subject by now that I wanted to dive right in, so I started out by learning about critical help through my Paramedical Science course whereby I believed would give me the right skills to move forward. Growing up I watched and took care of a family member that struggled in everyday life. Things so simple for someone healthy were not possible for this family member that suffered Chronic Obstructive Pulmonary Disease. This was now embedded into my upbringing and was the time in my life when I decided to pursue a profession that helps people, puts an end to these illnesses/diseases, and truly makes a difference in people's lives.

Due to this, I became increasingly interested in medicine over the years and since biology was always my favourite subject, at that moment I knew I wanted to pursue a medical career given my ambition and personal experiences. My favourite topics to study within biology were cell function, genetic mutation, the respiratory system and the nervous system. Another subject I also enjoyed was mathematics, especially the mechanics module, as this could be transferred to the human body structure, the skeleton. This made me appreciate the link between these subjects and another hobby of mine that a enjoy doing, ballet, whereby I understood the forces a body can generate, understood the anatomy of the body in order to know my limits, and understood why things are possible all while achieving my Advanced 2 from the Royal Academy of Dance. In addition to this, I also hold yoga classes whereby organisational and communicational skills are required. I enjoy making myself as well as helping others achieve their best self in mind, body and soul. In relation to hobbies and being outside of work, I have great enthusiasm for continuous learning whatever it may be. I have taken a Mental Health First Aid course. While trying to marry my passions of life, the outdoors and my medical background I always seem to find myself in hobbies which are linked to survival. I enjoy hiking, camping, canoeing, rock-climbing, navigating and stargazing. Once a week I instruct an indoor rock-climbing class, teaching people to correctly scale walls, overcome their fears in height and safely abseil down. All these hobbies have given me the leadership skills and confidence in my abilities to work with people in risky atmospheres when time management is of the essence.

The passion for medicine was later amplified when I experienced the compassion of the staff after I took a trip to the hospital following a compound leg fracture. The level of care I received that day stimulated my decision to enter the medical field by applying for a "NHS Hands-on Workshop". As my interest grew, so did my understanding and knowledge of the services I regard so highly. With my mind set, I involved myself in summer placements for work experience in order to observe all aspects of this grand system of processes (clinics, ward rounds, morgues, theatres, A&E problem solving, specialised treatments, on-calls & home visits), but most importantly I saw what it takes to be a good medical professional and how communication, much like many things in life, is the key to good patient-doctor relationships. I then signed up as a voluntary community first responder between my years while I planned my next phase of development and next steps of my road to becoming a successful doctor. I wanted to get an overall understanding of all types of medical roads via experiences before I went towards surgeon-based work experience as I believed this would further widen my knowledge and understanding of different scopes, therefore, I completed a research-based laboratory work experience which focussed work on developments towards lab-grown transplant tissue. Simultaneously, I would carry out self-organised education through books and mini courses. Once completed, I immediately managed to get myself onto a General Hospital placement where I followed the processes of local anaesthesia by shadowing a consultant. All these experiences had a striking feature in common, they were all fascinating and showed how medicine is almost a way of life. Understanding this was a key point for myself as theatre operations is all about teamwork. These experiences taught me how to problem solve, analyse situations, cooperate in a multidisciplinary environment and understand the attention to detail required.

I was taught on the importance of being calm, virtually meditating to mentally prepare yourself for the new experiences ahead, communicating and cooperation to your team, taking control of situations and being part of a force for the greater good. A vast amount of opportunities to learn existed, such as general surgery and trauma to knee, hip and arthroscopies whereby a plethora of techniques were available, for example seeing how a plate and screws would be fitted into a leg, which was intriguing due to the fact that I related to this from my past. I went on to observe other surgeries such as a tonsillectomy and an emergency surgery of a patient that had appendicitis. I wanted to further my educational experience, especially in the diagnosis area so I spent time with a Radiologist, studied X-Rays, MRI and CT scans in order to gather understanding of what pre-work is done before surgery. These lessons were inspirational as I too wanted to be part of a team that achieve these goals. In my time of experience, I covered many aspects of the field, which involved screening checks such as temperature and drug charts which could then lead to more in-situ checks such as wounds etc. This is where I appreciated the level of detail in the questions that need to be asked to patients. Again, the importance of communication kept reminding me how critical the doctor-patient relationship is. Before I pursued my goal of learning orthopaedics, I wanted to gain a deep insight into understanding the variations and importance of the anaesthetics applied so I shadowed the consultant over the course of many operations, from A&E and maternal aid to endoscopy and general surgery. Here I learnt that there are two mindsets, one for when performing planned surgery and one for when performing A&E surgery. Witnessing this was a real eye-opener as I felt the criticalness and urgency of the doctors while they also remained professional, efficient, unified and calm. Having no first-hand experience of this, I imagined myself in their shoes and instantly my heart rate began to rise and quickly realised that this is what I will be training for, this is what I will be doing to help people in need. My heart rate then began to drop as I continued to watch the surgery unfold.

While exploring different surgeries within this experience I now saw the constant and immense pressure medical staff face on a daily basis. This did not deter me, but in fact attracted me as I saw this as an opportunity for improvement and also understood that this pressure exists due to the reason that the line of work is one of most important in the world. Conversely, there will always be times when medical staff, including myself, may experience physical and emotional stresses that are imposed within the theatre. Here, it was revealed to me of what personal and work sacrifices need to be made in order to best treat patients. Throughout these experiences I took advantage of my medical degree as much as possible to help me get a deeper understanding and interaction of situations. I then decided to gain educational exposure in post mortems by actively participating. This is when I realised the medical path is one with endless learning and countless life-long possibilities. A profession so rich in knowledge is one that will keep all those devoted to it continuously improving, developing and satisfying that thirst for knowledge. These demonstrations to which I took part in highlighted the realistic impressions and expectations of what it means to be a medical professional. While completing these programs, I understood that there are numerous of improvements that should be made within our system as a whole. Medical staff gets exposed to large amounts of stress due to the nature of the job and the system, and processes that define it, should be made as smooth as possible to minimise additional issues that may occur. For this reason, I decided to enrol and complete a Local Leadership program in hope that I can make a positive difference for the future.

I have always enjoyed teaching, leading and guiding people/ children, teaching them skills such as swimming, reading, writing and basketball which all taught me the patience needed and the appreciation of everyone's uniqueness. In addition to teaching activities, I would also teach mathematics to younger students as tuition as well as run the scouts. After a while you pick up on what works best for individuals and teach everyone differently, especially when individuals require special attention due to conditions. I have learnt to appreciate life so much more and approach it as well as others with a warm and caring nature. Some of the people were also foreign and would struggle to communicate, so I took it upon myself to try and learn as much of their language as possible. Even now I am still learning Spanish to improve my ability to communicate to a wider audience. This way I want to approach the medical system. I would love to be given the opportunity to improve on what we have by listening to people's problems, both patients and doctors alike. However, the only way I can achieve this is through doing what I would love to do, and that is being a doctor myself. I am confident that I can make a difference all while getting that job satisfaction.

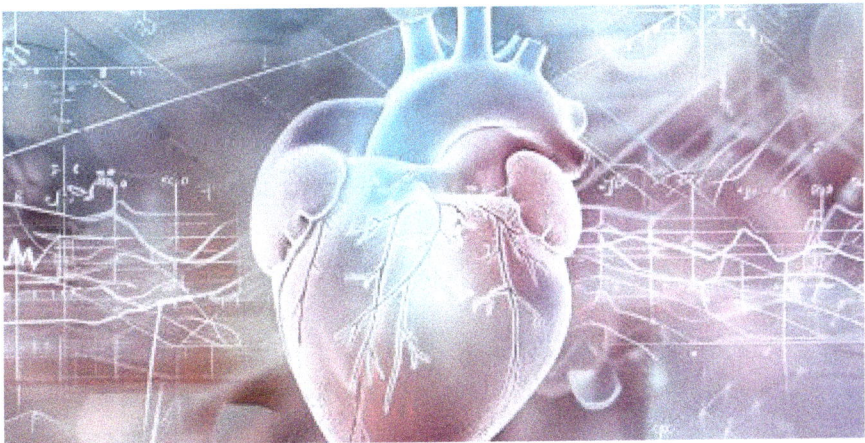

All the above experiences helped me understand the complex yet rewarding career a medical professional can have. Now knowing at least part of what it takes to follow my desire and become a medical professional, I can say that I also know and understand that I definitely want to pursue this and put my skills to the test as well as allow them to grow. Balancing the above has been critical for maintaining my continuous improvement and involvement in various activities in addition to my experiences. For this reason, I believe I am a professional, reliable and enthusiastic individual while having the ability of gaining deeper involvement due to my scientific background and work classes I have carried out through hobbies or interests. I believe with my communications skills, drive of ambition, analytical and problem-solving nature I can be a valuable asset to the institution, ultimately driving positive change, serving medicine and its people, improvement of people's health and becoming a professional practitioner of this art. I look forward to pursuing this inspirational vocation with excitement, opening many doors all with evermore knowledge and ways to help people in need. This will definitely be a challenge, but it is one that I seek and would take over and over again every time as I know the rewards of fulfilment and gratification are limitless.

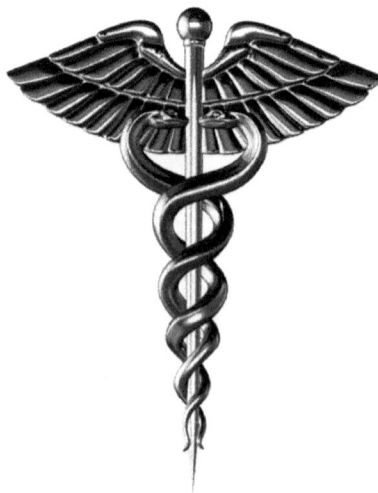

6.10 Interview Process & Tips

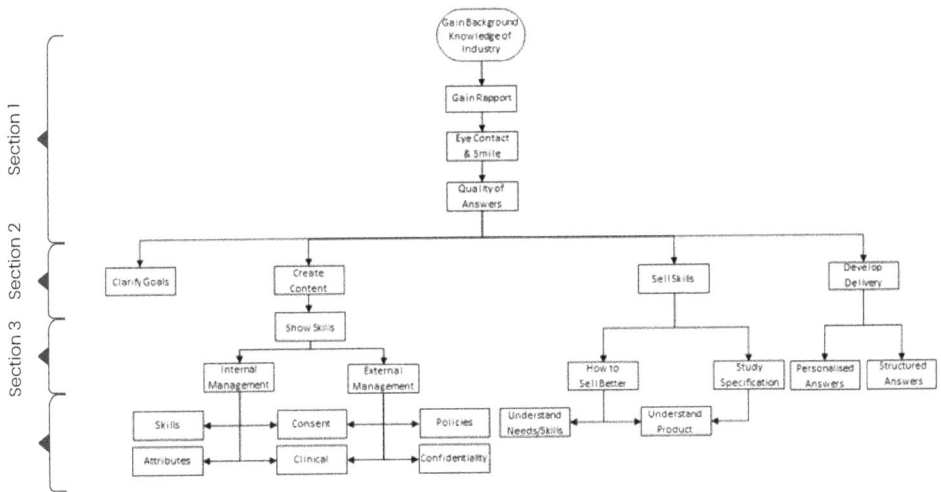

Fig.1- Interview Process

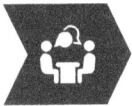

Section 1: Main interview steps consist of 4 key areas; Strengthen these areas in order to succeed. Know what your talking about, talk about it with flow, talk in a way that is interactive, and give them the quality answers.

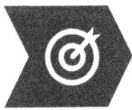

Section 2: Answers should include these essential tips; Clarify your goals, create your content, make your content attractive and valuable in order to sell your skills, and delivery your content in a desirable manner.

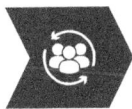

Section 3: Having taken the above tips into account, these areas within Section 3 will be topics that you will need to explore and engage the panel with your answers.

1. Firstly, you will need to talk about your personal and internal management, or how you manage externally towards others. This is how you will show your skills as a person and how others will perceive you. This will help the panel decide whether or not you will be good to work with. The content you create in your answers must include the above. A lot of the time interviewers want to know how you did something, not what you actually did.

2. Secondly, you will need to know how to sell your skills by knowing how to better sell yourself in general. Having studied the specification of the job/role and what the requirements are will aid in this.

3. Thirdly, as you create your content to show your skills and sell your skills you will need to ensure that the content you are creating is deliverable and easily digested (excuse the medical pun). The only way to have a positive impact in content delivery is to make things personal, real, structured and simple. This works for a lot of things in life.

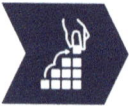

Section 4: Lastly, this fundamental knowledge as well as these traits are required to form the basis of all the above sections. This is the core that will shape everything. Pay attention to this section and the rest will fall into place. Show your skills, attributes, professionalism, confidentiality, clinical knowledge and ethical attitude regarding consent and adherence to policies. Understand everyone's needs, this includes the patient's, your department's and your own. Know your skills, and understand what you are really trying to achieve as a service. This is your product.

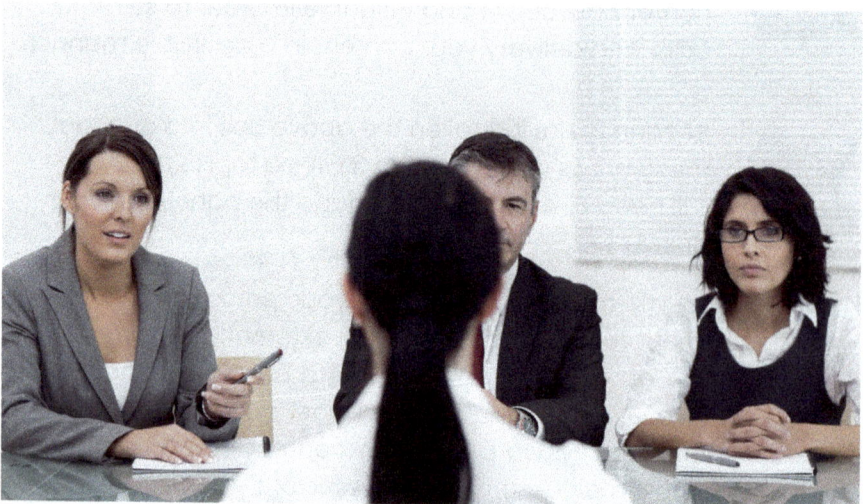

EPILOGUE

Concluding this comprehensive guide, it's essential to reflect on the journey you are called to embark on towards becoming a health professional with clear understanding. This is more than just a manual; it's a testament to the values, dedication, and resilience required to succeed in the medical field. The book it is meticulously outlining the intricacies of preparing for and excelling in your medical/healthcare career journey, highlighting the profound impact of knowledge, preparation, and personal integrity.

Throughout this, it is delved into the fundamental qualities that define a successful doctor/health professional: compassion, communication, dedication, and continuous self-improvement. These attributes are not just theoretical concepts but practical skills and attitudes that will shape your professional life and personal growth. The emphasis on understanding oneself, preparing thoroughly for the challenges ahead, and maintaining a commitment to ethical practice and patient care forms the backbone of this guide.

In the ever-evolving landscape of healthcare, where technology and human interaction intertwine, it is your passion for science and humanity that will guide you. The detailed steps provided for interviews and career preparation are designed to equip you with the tools needed to present yourself effectively and genuinely. Remember, every interaction is an opportunity to demonstrate your commitment to the medical profession and your willingness to learn and adapt.

As you move forward, keep In mind the core values discussed. Strive to be empathetic, patient, and resilient. Embrace the continuous learning process, and never underestimate the power of a kind word or a compassionate gesture. Your journey in medicine is not just about achieving professional milestones but also about making a meaningful difference in the lives of others.

Read the examples that are written and adapt them according to your experiences. These are only indicators of how people could prepare themselves.

The world needs dedicated health professionals who are not only skilled but also deeply human. By adhering to the principles and advice laid out in this guide, you are not just preparing for a career; you are preparing to join a noble tradition of individuals who are committed to healing, supporting, and advancing the well-being of humanity.

In the book it is mentioned the phrase, "Go for it!", and by using it someone has to understand that needs to be equipped with knowledge, remain steadfast in their values, and embrace the journey with enthusiasm and be flexible and decisive to the goal but also to be courageous and concur the future obstacles without fear but with determination. The road ahead may be challenging, but with the right preparation and mindset, you are destined to make a lasting impact in the field of medicine/health care.

May your path be filled with learning, growth, and the profound satisfaction that comes from serving others. The future of healthcare is bright, and it holds endless possibilities for those who are prepared, compassionate, and driven to excel.

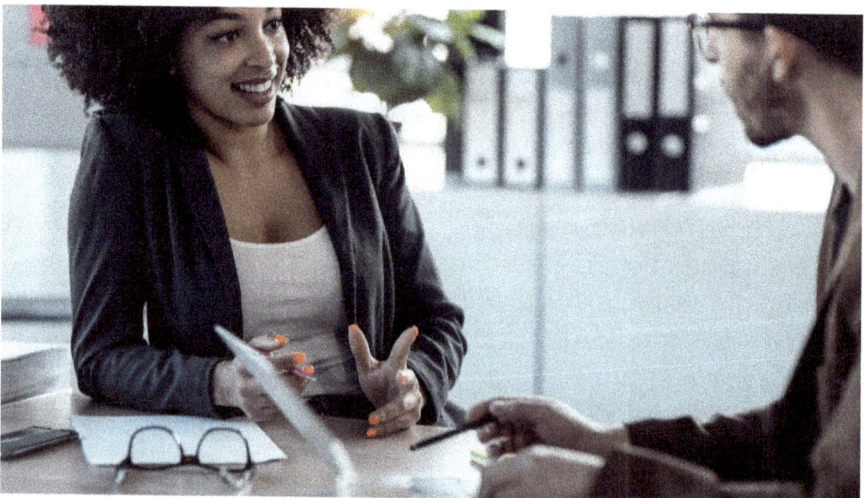

BIOGRAPHY

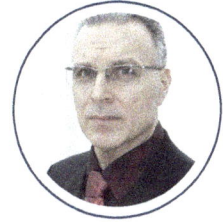

Professor George Zafiropoulos is a Senior Consultant Orthopaedic Surgeon that is actively involved in Medical Education, lecturing in universities and continues to practice his profession while constantly keeping up to date with the advances. He has vast experience in managing departments, leading teams and research projects, coaching students and junior doctors, greatly impacting their development while giving them advice for their future careers and overlooking their progress. His abundance of knowledge and understanding allows him to offer his mentored students a head start in their careers as there is more to a professional medical occupation than just skill. His approach has enabled departments to grow and prosper as his work is adopted by departments not only his own, thus building and improving on systems as a whole. His work has reached many parts of the world but has also practised medicine in numerous global locations to continuously improve organisations and positively impact patients' lives. Being a member of numerous interview panels, his medical experience and opinion on interview techniques is internationally respected and practised by his own students who go on to achieve positive and successful careers.

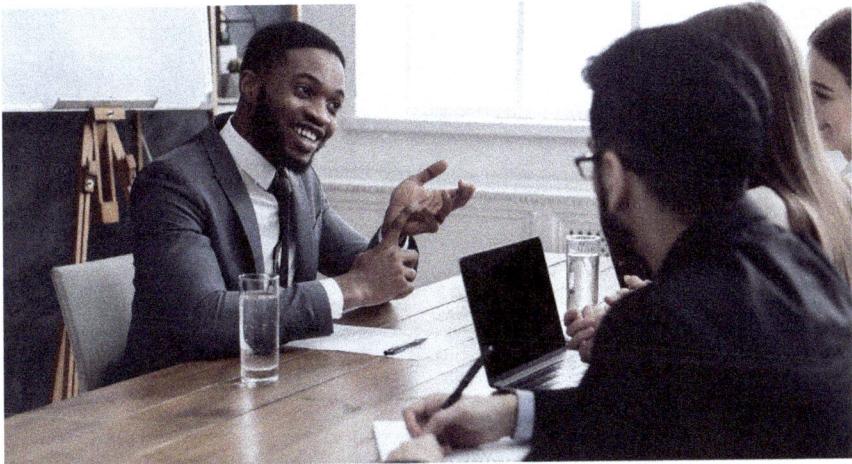

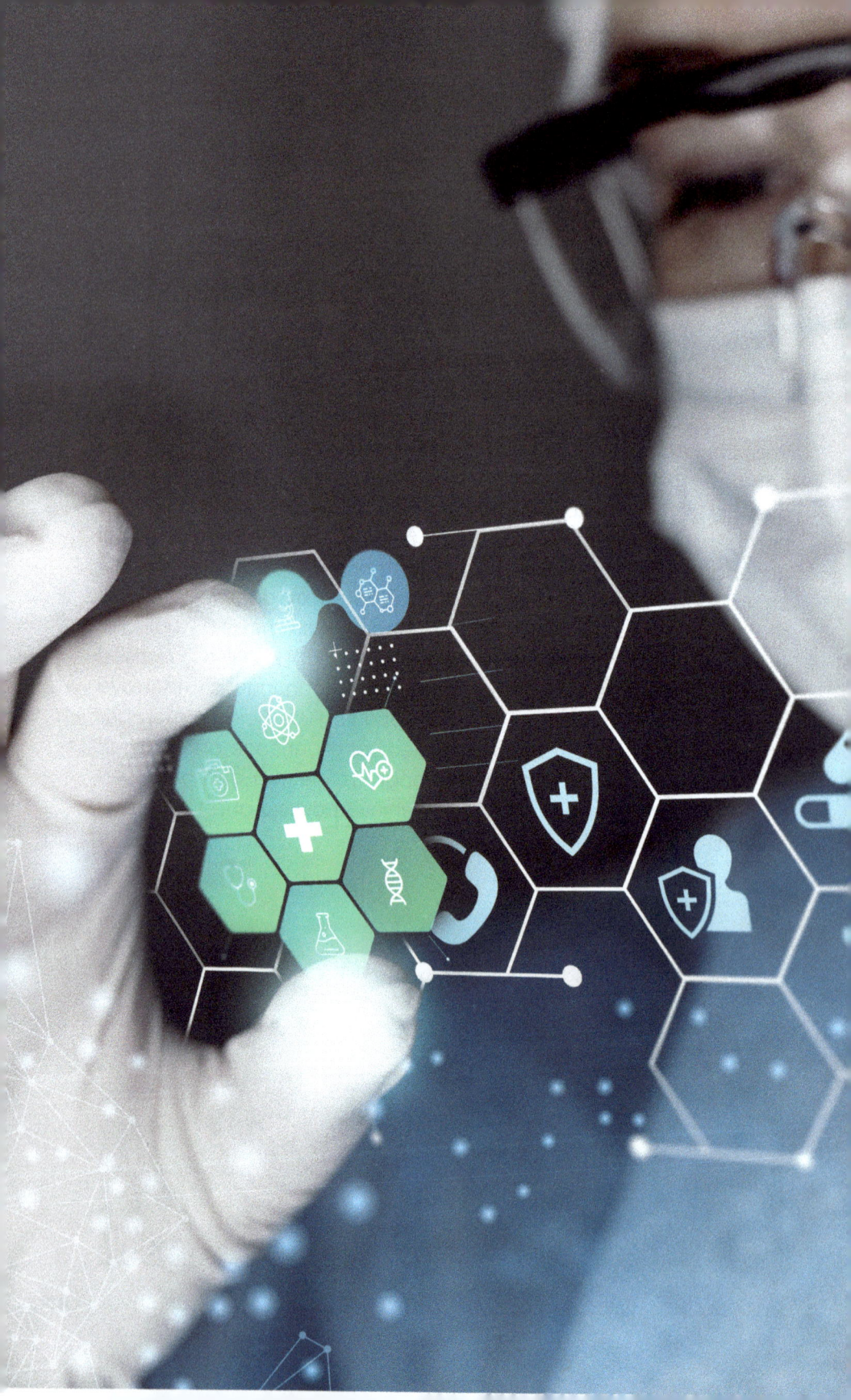

www.ingramcontent.com/pod-product-compliance
Lightning Source LLC
Chambersburg PA
CBHW071440210326
41597CB00020B/3877